Fast Facts in Childhood Poisoning

Fast Facts in Childhood Poisoning

Sumitha Nayak
MD DNB PGDMLS PGDGC
Consultant Pediatrician
The Children's Clinic
Bengaluru, Karnataka, India

Foreword

Padmaja Aradhya

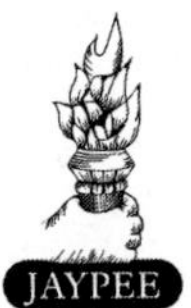

JAYPEE BROTHERS MEDICAL PUBLISHERS
The Health Sciences Publisher
New Delhi | London

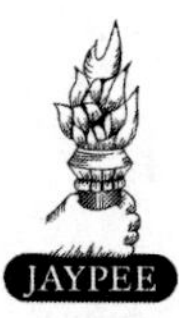

Jaypee Brothers Medical Publishers (P) Ltd

Headquarters
EMCA House
23/23-B, Ansari Road, Daryaganj
New Delhi - 110 002, India
Landline: +91-11-23272143, +91-11-23272703
+91-11-23282021, +91-11-23245672
E-mail: jaypee@jaypeebrothers.com

Corporate Office
4838/24, Ansari Road, Daryaganj
New Delhi - 110 002, India
Phone: +91-11-43574357
Fax: +91-11-43574314
E-mail: jaypee@jaypeebrothers.com

Overseas Office
J.P. Medical Ltd
83 Victoria Street, London
SW1H 0HW (UK)
Phone: +44 20 3170 8910
E-mail: info@jpmedpub.com

EU GPSR Authorised Representative
Logos Europe, 9 rue Nicolas Poussin
17000, La Rochelle, France
Phone: +33 (0) 6 67 93 73 78
E-mail: contact@logoseurope.eu

Website: www.jaypeebrothers.com
Website: www.jaypeedigital.com

Inquiries for bulk sales may be solicited at: jaypee@jaypeebrothers.com

Fast Facts in Childhood Poisoning

First Edition: 2013, Reprint: **2026**

ISBN 978-93-5090-632-3

Printed at: Samrat Offset Pvt. Ltd.

Dedicated to

All my little patients who have helped me, through the years, to hone my skills as a pediatrician.

All my teachers, who taught me the skills of pediatrics.

My close friends and colleagues, who have inspired me to attempt to reach higher goals.

Above all, my family, who has stood behind me always, in all my endeavors and constantly encouraged me to reach for the stars.

Foreword

Common poisons available in households differ according to the nationalities. They depend on the culture, economic status, beliefs and needs of the people. Therefore, poison control policies need to be designed according to cultural and societal requirements. Here in the United States of America, poison control to a large extent, has been easier as there is a centralized poison control center where we can make a phone call and read out the label of whatever the child has consumed and we will be guided through with appropriate management. Unfortunately, in India there is no such centralized poison control.

Dr Sumitha Nayak has written this book, which would be of great help to physicians who are managing childhood poisonings in their clinics and hospitals. For instance, kerosene oil, which is available in almost every home, can be consumed by a child, the management of which can be difficult for, say, a pediatrician in Greece or any other country. This book offers management of such incidences and will give a quick reference and treatment and help avoid long-term complications. Organophosphorus compounds can be very dangerous in any patient, pediatric or adult. To recognize even the symptoms of organophosphorus compounds can be quite formidable and daunting if you do not know what to look for. Every Indian physician is aware of scorpion bites and snake bites, which are common in India and the management of which can be very difficult without knowing exactly what to look for. This book will be quite handy and helpful in the exercise and control of such incidences. Drugs like tricyclic antidepressant can affect the cardiovascular system and the management of which becomes not only urgent, but also life saving. Every pediatrician is aware of lead poisoning, which can result in encephalopathy in young kids. Recognition of these common, but lethal incidences can lead to a better outcome for the patients and make for a better physician. Last, but not least, the medications, which are commonly kept at home, like paracetamol and non-steroidal anti-inflammatory drugs can be quite dangerous in young children even when taken in small quantities.

I am writing a foreword for my good friend, Dr Sumitha Nayak for the second time and I wish her all the best in her endeavors. This is a very valuable book and I hope to see a lot more books by her, which would be of practical use to the physician community worldwide.

Padmaja Aradhya MD
[Diplomate American Board of Psychiatry and Neurology (Neurology), Diplomate American Board of Electrodiagnostic Medicine, Diplomate American Board of Psychiatry and Neurology (Neuromuscular Medicine), Diplomate American Board of Psychiatry and Neurology (Vascular Neurology)]
4230 Hempstead Turnpike
Suite 106, Bethpage, NY 11714, USA
E-mail: paradhya@yahoo.com

Preface

Fast Facts in Childhood Poisoning is a concise book covering all aspects of childhood poisonings. This book was conceptualized when, as a postgraduate student, I was faced with the daunting task of handling poison cases, in an emergency situation, with no time to open the large textbooks to check every step in the management of the patient. I felt the need for a handy book, which could be easily carried in the coat pocket and which would act as an immediate guide for all the needs of the case, in terms of investigations to be done, emergency management and definitive management, specific antidotes and as well as follow-up care. In short, the book must provide comprehensive and current information on the management of poison cases.

This book has attempted to cover all the needs in a convenient and easy to follow format, with tables, diagrams and algorithms and wherever indicated mnemonics for easy recall. It also covers topics related to prevention of poisoning, counseling for prevention of poisoning and follow-up care. Extensive research has ensured current management and standard international practices for every topic.

It is an invaluable book for all pediatricians, intensivists, physicians and students who handle cases of poisoning in children.

Sumitha Nayak

Preface

Acknowledgments

My deep gratitude to Prakash, my dear husband, who has given me unconditional support through all my trials in life and has always encouraged me to follow my dreams and reach for the stars.

Nikhil and Nishant, my dearest and loving sons, who have always been my best critics and have assisted me whenever I have faltered in the use of technology.

To my family, dear friends and well-wishers who have spared their valuable time and encouraged me with their good wishes.

And above all, to my beloved parents, who taught me to stand on my feet and always encouraged me to stretch out and reach for the impossible.

Contents

Section III: Warfare

Section IV: Venoms

Section V: Miscellaneous

Section VI: Preventive Measures

I

Section

General Principles

1 Chapter — General Principles for Treatment of Childhood Poisoning

Toxin ingestion may be intentional, especially in teenagers and adolescents or accidental in toddlers and younger children. Intentional ingestion is usually with multiple substances, hence the signs and symptoms may not be typical of any particular substance. It could also vary depending on whether it was consumed on an empty stomach or after food, as absorption can vary when there is food in the stomach. Also, the hyperactive children, those with pre-existing neurological problems and those with pre-existing diseases, may show exaggerated signs.

INITIAL ASSESSMENT

When a child with a suspected poisoning is brought in, it is essential to first stabilize the patient and then attempt to find out what poison had been ingested. Take into consideration all the possible substances, over-the-counter (OTC) medications and drugs that could have been brought in by any visitors to the home. All medications should be seen, preferably in the original containers or packs. The type of poison, agents and specific antidotes are given in Table 1.1.

Emergency Stabilization of the Patient

Check and Stabilize

1. Airway: Ensure that the airway is clear and clean, free from any ingested matter, vomitus of other obstructions. If essential, place a mouth gag to prevent damage to the tongue and teeth.
2. Breathing: Ensure that the patient is breathing comfortably. Administer supplemental oxygen to ensure adequate tissue perfusion.

Table 1.1: Specific antidotes

Type of poison	Agent	Antidote
Acetaminophen	Acetaminophen	N-acetylcysteine
Anticoagulant	Warfarin, rat poison	Vitamin K
Cardiac drugs	Beta blockers, digoxin, calcium channel blockers	Calcium chloride, glucagon
Cholinergic—muscarinic, nicotinic	Organophosphates, some mushrooms	Atropine, Pralidoxime
Ethylene glycol	Antifreeze	Ethanol
Hydrogen sulfide	Industrial gas leaks	Sodium nitrite
Iron	Iron containing products	Deferoxamine
Opioid	Opioid	Naloxone
Lead	Lead containing products	Dimercaptosuccinic acid (DMSA), D-penicillamine
Mercury	Mercury containing products	DMSA, British anti-Lewisite (BAL), D-penicillamine
Naphtha	Napthalene balls	Methylene blue
Arsenic	Arsenic compounds, contaminated fish	BAL, DMSA

3. Circulatory status to be noted. Intravenous (IV) access to be obtained immediately, to facilitate administration of fluids and drugs before circulatory collapse or compromise occurs.
4. Obtain a random blood sugar level, especially in those who have altered mental status or with signs of hypoglycemia. When the blood sugar level is lower than 80 mg/dL (4.4 mmol/L), it is essential to administer IV glucose rapidly to reverse the signs.

   Dose: Infants: 5 mL/kg of 10% dextrose.

   Children: 4 mL/kg of 25% dextrose.
5. Intravenous thiamine is recommended to be administered, before the dextrose infusion, to prevent the occurrence of Wernicke's encephalopathy.

   Dose: Infants: 10 mg.

   Children: 10–25 mg.

6. Pulse oximetry, especially in those with altered mental status will help to guide the oxygen supplementation that has to be administered.
7. Electrocardiogram (ECG) in all leads is essential as a baseline, before the start of cardiac monitoring. It also gives information regarding any cardiotoxic effects of the ingested substance.
8. Watch out for 'toxidromes' the symptoms that could point to particular toxin exposure. Observe the breath for any characteristic odors, which can lead to a diagnosis about the toxin.
9. Removal of the poison—if it is present around the mouth, on the skin or as vomitus, it must be washed out with copious water and all external traces of the poison must be removed.

Points to Note

1. The typical textbook presentations of each toxicity may not be present in every patient. Hence, a strong index of suspicion is essential to make an accurate diagnosis and successful treatment of the patient.
2. Adolescents and older children who have intentionally consumed poisons, usually take a combination of substances. Here, again the presentations vary and poses a challenge for diagnosis.
3. Every child who has consumed a toxin, whether accidentally or intentionally needs to be counseled and closely monitored after recovery, so that there is no repetition, as well as any associated or underlying comorbidities are corrected at the earliest.
4. Ensure that all persons who are closely associated with the child, especially the immediate family are made aware of the seriousness of the situation and cooperate to ensure that the child is not exposed to the toxins again.
5. Counseling of the parents and family members is essential to sensitize them to the gravity of the issue at hand.
6. Wherever possible, use of childproof or tamper-proof medicine bottles, is to be encouraged. Parents and caregivers are encouraged to keep their medications out of reach of children, especially the toddlers.

7. Parents must never administer medications to the child by telling them, it is a candy or a sweet, which makes the younger children desire to consume it in larger quantities.

Laboratory Tests

Tests will help to corroborate the clinical diagnosis, while at the same time, assess the patient's clinical status during the course of stay in the hospital (Table 1.2).

Table 1.2: Different laboratory tests to corroborate clinical diagnosis

Laboratory tests	Clinical diagnosis
Blood glucose	Ingestion of hypoglycemic agents
Serum bicarbonate	Renal failure Acidosis
Serum electrolyte	Electrolyte imbalance Renal failure
Pulse oximetry	Hypoxia
ECG in all leads	Cardiotoxicity
Prothrombin time, coagulation profile	Coagulopathy
Urinalysis	Renal failure
Arterial blood gas	Hypoxemia
Urine drug screen	Specific drug ingestion

Supportive Treatment

The treatment of poisonings in children follow confirmed and time-tested patterns, with the recommendations for induced emesis and gastric decontamination forming the basis of therapy. However, nowadays, the role of induced emesis is limited, as it has not been found to improve the patient outcome. The use of emetics like syrup of ipecac has been long abandoned by the American Academy of Pediatrics, as well as the European and American Toxicology Committees. It has not been found to improve the patient's condition, even if administered within few minutes of toxin consumption.

Gastric Decontamination

Gastric lavage has been used as the method to remove the ingested toxins from the stomach. It has maximal benefits, when it is done as soon as possible, generally within 1 hour after toxin ingestion. A relatively large bore orogastric tube is inserted and normal saline is administered. The contents are withdrawn immediately using a large syringe and the input must match the output. The wash is usually continued, until the solution is clear. The risks associated with gastric lavage are:

- Esophageal trauma
- Laryngeal trauma
- Aspiration
- Nausea, vomiting
- Impairment of the level of consciousness.

Contraindications to gastric lavage are illustrated in Figure 1.1.

Adsorption Agents

Activated charcoal is used to decrease the absorption of ingested toxins from the stomach. It is useful in cases of poisoning with dapsone, phenobarbital, theophylline, salicylates, phenytoin, valproic acid, carbamazepine or quinine.

Activated charcoal acts by decreasing the enterohepatic and the enteroenteric recirculation of the ingested drugs, which usually occurs in the gut lumen. However, not all the drugs are well adsorbed by this agent and hence, it's usefulness may be limited in children. The color and consistency are other deterrents in their usefulness in childhood poisonings.

When indicated, it is recommended to administer activated charcoal as soon as possible after toxin ingestion, preferably within 1 hour. The first dose is generally administered along with sorbitol, which improves the taste, as well as the transit through the gastrointestinal tract (GIT), as it is a cathartic agent. Subsequent doses do not need to be administered along with sorbitol as it can give rise to severe fluid and electrolyte imbalances.

Dose recommended in children: 1–2 g/kg body weight, in cases of unknown quantity of drug ingestion. When the ingested amount can be determined, a 10:1 charcoal-drug ratio needs to be administered for the desired effects.

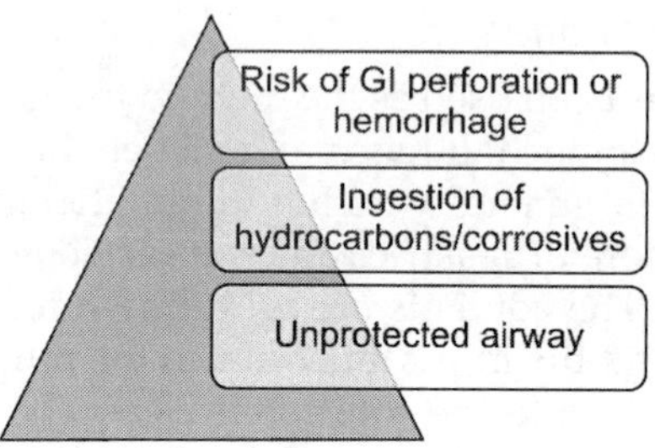

Fig. 1.1: Contraindications to gastric lavage (GI, gastrointestinal)

Cathartics

Cathartics are administered with the presumption that they can aid the movement of the toxic agent through the GIT and hence assist in the excretion from the system. However, the role of cathartics in children is doubtful due to the risk of electrolyte and fluid imbalances, which can cause major complications to the existing toxicity. Sorbitol is a cathartic, which is usually used along with the initial dose of activated charcoal in a dose of 1–2 g/kg body weight.

Polyethylene glycol is another cathartic agent, which is used for whole bowel irrigation following toxicity. It is used in cases of poisoning with sustained release drug preparations or in case of heavy metal toxicity. However, it has a limited role in childhood poisoning.

Emetics

Following the ingestion of toxins, the attempt used to be made to expel the toxin by inducing vomiting, in an attempt to decrease the amount of ingested toxin. However, the administration of emetic agents like syrup of ipecac is no longer recommended, as it has not been found to produce any beneficial effects in children, but may pose a danger of aspiration in case of unprotected airways.

Urine Alkalinization and Hemodialysis

Excretion of certain toxins can be accelerated via the urinary route. In these cases, by changing the urine pH, it is possible to aid the drug excretion. For example, methotrexate, etc.

Urinary alkalinization is useful in cases of toxicity with salicylates, tricyclic antidepressants, phenobarbital. This is done by administering IV fluids, usually half normal saline to which 50–150 mEq of sodium bicarbonate has been added per liter, to result in an isotonic fluid. The rate of administration is 1–2 L/h. After adequate urine output has been established, KCl is added in a dose of 20–40 mEq/L. The urine pH must be maintained from 7.5 to 8.5.

Hemodialysis involves the circulation of the blood through an extracorporeal membrane and is indicated in cases, where the patient's condition is rapidly deteriorating when the endogenous clearance of the drug is low or when massive amounts of drug ingestion has taken place.

Hemodialysis is useful in cases of toxicity with salicylates, theophylline, phenobarbital, methanol or valproic acid.

Hemoperfusion involves the passage of the blood through an extracorporeal membrane, which contains an adsorbent like activated charcoal or polystyrene resin. As the thin membrane has a larger surface area, there is more drug adhesion and excretion from the circulation.

SUGGESTED READING

1. Kleigman RM, Behrman RE, Jenson HB, et al. Nelson Textbook of Pediatrics, 18th edition. Elsevier Health Sciences Division; 2007.
2. McGregor T, Parkar M, Roa S. Evaluation and management of common childhood poisonings. Am Fam Physician. 2009 Mar;79(5):397-403.

II

Section

Chemical Poisoning

2 Chapter Hydrocarbons

KEROSENE OIL

KEROSENE POISONING IN CHILDREN

Kerosene is a liquid hydrocarbon mixture, which is a byproduct of the distillation of crude oil. It is used extensively as a alternative source of energy and is used for cooking food especially in the remote areas. Accidental ingestion of kerosene oil is a common problem, especially in the hot summer months when the liquid is mistakenly ingested, especially by children when they find the containers lying within easy reach. Intentional ingestion may occur in older children and adolescents with suicidal intention or as substance abuse.

Pathophysiology

Toxicity caused by kerosene is via inhalation of the fumes during ingestion. Dermal absorption may occasionally occur, when the liquid is accidentally spilled off in cases or immersion of the limbs or body in the liquid, which is a rare occurrence. Aspiration of the fumes causes substantial damage to the lung tissues. Kerosene vapor has a low volatility due to which it causes chemical pneumonitis in the lung parenchyma. It causes morphological changes in the tracheal epithelium and may also cause cardiovascular changes similar to atherosclerosis. The volatile chemicals can displace alveolar oxygen and cause hypoxia. Direct contact with the alveolar epithelium can cause hemorrhage, hypoxia, edema, inactivation of the surfactant and vascular thrombosis. Dermal absorption of the kerosene liquid over a period of time can result in erythema and dermatitis, which is due to the chemical irritation. It could cause local necrosis, followed by tissue regeneration, which can be repetitive in cases of prolonged or recurrent exposures.

Symptoms

Kerosene has a bad taste hence, large volumes are rarely ingested; usually not more than 30 mL is consumed by children, commonly a few drops. The symptoms can begin within 30 minutes after consumption and progress during the first 24–48 hours and subside after 1–2 weeks. In children, the respiratory symptoms are prolonged.

Respiratory symptoms: Usually begin within a few hours after exposure. The child may present with cough, difficulty in breathing and tightness in the chest, choking, grunting and tachypnea.

Gastrointestinal tract (GIT): Irritation can cause abdominal pain and nausea. Vomiting may occur and would increase the likelihood of pulmonary aspiration.

Central nervous system (CNS): Toxic effects like depression, disinhibition and euphoria, similar to that of narcotic poisoning, may be manifested. Subsequently the patient may complain of lethargy, headache and obtundation. Occasionally seizures may occur, which is usually secondary to hypoxia.

Signs

1. Respiratory signs are commonly observed. Tachypnea, grunting, cyanosis, rales and wheezing may be found.
2. Central nervous system: Dizziness, lethargy, ataxia, seizures, coma.
3. Gastrointestinal tract: Persistent vomiting, abdominal pain.
4. Cardiovascular system: Cardiac arrhythmias, which can cause sudden death.
5. Cutaneous: Mucosal irritation.
6. Chemical skin burns.

Investigations

1. Pulse oximetry: It will give an estimate of the hypoxia due to the kerosene ingestion.
2. Arterial blood gas (ABG):
    i. Estimates accurately the extent of hypoxemia in severely affected patients.

ii. Hypercarbia may be observed secondary to respiratory depression and decreased pulmonary gas exchange.

3. Serum electrolytes: Usually in the normal range. Increased anion gap may indicate the coingestion of another toxic substance.
4. X-ray of the chest: It is essential, especially in all the symptomatic children. Initial X-rays may not show any abnormality, but progression may occur over time. Common abnormality noted is basal infiltrates of the lungs. Other findings include perihilar opacities and atelectasis. Repeat chest X-rays need to be taken to note any progression or changes like pneumothorax or pneumomediastinum that may develop later. In case of asymptomatic children, it is essential to repeat the chest X-ray after 6 hours to document the negative findings or to note any progression.
5. Electrocardiogram (ECG): In all leads to identify any dysrhythmias that may occur in the patient.

Treatment

1. Decontaminate the child. Remove the child from the environs of the kerosene oil, change the clothes and wash the skin with soap and water. This reduces the further absorption of the toxic vapors of kerosene.
2. Never induce emesis in the patient who has consumed kerosene, as this worsens the chances of aspiration.
3. Stabilize the patient, administer supplemental oxygen. Early intubation and ventilation may be occasionally indicated.
4. Ensure the airway is open and insert the venous access line.
5. Gastric decontamination by lavage is not advised, as the amount of kerosene ingested is usually minimal.
6. Treatment with prophylactic antibiotics is not indicated, unless the patient has definite evidence of pulmonary involvement.
7. In case of severe respiratory distress or depressed level of consciousness, the patient needs to be intubated and adequately ventilated with positive end-expiratory pressure ventilation.

Complications

1. Aspiration pneumonitis.
2. Pneumothorax.
3. Pneumatocele.
4. Seizures.
5. Encephalopathy.
6. Memory loss.
7. Myocarditis.
8. Cardiomyopathy.

Prognosis

With early and appropriate supportive care, complete recovery usually occurs. Radiological recovery occurs later than clinical recovery.

NAPHTHALENE

NAPHTHALENE POISONING IN CHILDREN

Naphthalene balls are used as moth repellents to keep the woolen and other clothes insect free. They are available in the form of small white balls, which can be easily slipped into corners. The naphthalene balls have an aromatic odor and appear attractive to children.

Naphthalene is a bicyclic aromatic compound, which is a hydrocarbon and it vaporizes easily giving a pungent and characteristic smell.

Naphthalene toxicity is usually accidental in children, but can be intentional in older children and adolescents. In children suffering from glucose-6-phosphate dehydrogenase (G6PD) deficiency, the effects of naphthalene toxicity are extremely severe and could be life-threatening.

How can people be exposed to naphthalene?

People could be exposed to naphthalene through:

1. Breathing low levels in outdoor air. People could breathe it from a factory release or if they work, where moth repellents, coal tar products, dyes or inks are produced. Exposure can also happen from breathing smoke from burning wood, tobacco, coal or natural gas.
2. Consumption of drinking water with naphthalene in it. Eating foods or beverages with naphthalene is unlikely.
3. Touching fabrics treated with moth repellents containing naphthalene.
4. Eye contact by getting naphthalene in the eyes from vapors or by touching eyes with contaminated hands.

Toxic dose: Not known in children. Even one mothball ingested can result toxicity in children.

Pathophysiology

When naphthalene enters the body through any one of the above mentioned routes, it enters the bloodstream. Due to the lipid peroxidation, it induces RBC hemolysis, which is pronounced in those who are unable to withstand oxidative stress, like G6PD patients and carriers. The massive hemolysis results in anemia, jaundice and hemoglobinuria. Methemoglobinemia results from the conversion of the ferrous to ferric hemoglobin. Cyanosis can result due to the decreased oxygen carrying capacity of the hemoglobin. Renal failure can occur due to the massive hemoglobinuria. Most of the naphthalene is excreted by the body in 3–4 days.

Symptoms

Non-specific symptoms may occur:

- Nausea, vomiting, abdominal pain
- Restlessness, fever, headache
- Sweating, confusion
- Painful micturition
- Difficulty in breathing.

Signs

- Fever
- Anemia
- Tachycardia
- Hypotension
- Hyperkalemia
- Icterus
- Hematuria
- Convulsions
- Altered sensorium.

Investigations

1. Hemoglobin levels to be estimated, to give an idea regarding the extent of hemolysis.
2. Urine exam—presence of hemoglobinuria will be noted.
3. Liver function tests—extent of liver function impairment, elevated bilirubin and transaminases.
4. Peripheral smear—shows evidence of hemolysis, Heinz bodies.
5. Pulse oximetry—shows the saturation. However, with associated methemoglobinemia, the pulse oximeter readings may not be indicative of the actual saturation.

6. ABG, which measures the arterial PO_2. In case of associated methemoglobinemia, the PO_2 levels could be normal. Hence, clinical suspicion is essential.

   When the cyanosis is not responding to high levels of free-flow oxygen, in the absence of cardiorespiratory causes, always suspect methemoglobinemia.
7. Serum potassium levels—may show hyperkalemia.
8. Serum and urine levels of naphthalene—elevated levels indicative of toxicity.

Treatment

Supportive Treatment

1. Remove the clothes and wash the exposed parts, skin or eyes.
2. Maintain the airway patency.
3. Administer oxygen and ensure that patient is breathing spontaneously and adequately. In case patient is in altered sensorium, intubate and ventilate the patient.
4. Maintain adequate circulation, place the IV line and administer IV fluids. In case of hypotension, run the fluids rapidly at 20 mL/kg in the 1st hour, till the hypotension is corrected. Adequate hydration is also essential to ensure urinary elimination of the toxin.
5. In case patient has arrived early, gastric decontamination may be attempted. Administer activated charcoal to adsorb the naphthalene.

Specific Treatment

1. Intravenous methylene blue is the antidote to treat the methemoglobinemia. Administer at the rate of 1.5 mg/kg intravenously.
2. Packed RBC transfusion can be administered depending on the level of the anemia. In case of ongoing hemolysis, repeated RBC transfusions may be required.
3. Oral ascorbic acid 300 mg/day will help to decrease the methemoglobinemia.
4. N-acetylcysteine is also used to decrease the methemoglobinemia, especially in G6PD patients who may not tolerate the methylene blue treatment.

5. Continuous venovenous hemofiltration to maintain continuous elimination of the toxins. It is superior to hemodialysis, as in the presence of continued hemolysis, the toxin elimination must be maintained for adequate recovery to occur.

Complications

Naphthalene balls can remain in the stomach and continue to exert delayed symptoms and continued hemolysis.

TURPENTINE

TURPENTINE POISONING IN CHILDREN

Turpentine is a hydrocarbon, belonging to the group of terpenes, which are natural products that have medicinal properties and biological activity. It is obtained for distillation of some ingredients of pine trees. They may be present in cleaning agents besides being used as rubefacients and in aromatherapy. It may also be present in wax polishes, floor polish and in brush cleaners.

Turpentine or turpentine oil is liquid with a pungent odor and hence, is not very palatable. Usually, accidental ingestion may occur when the container is mistakenly opened. Some cultures use turpentine as a purgative, anthelmintic and as a general elixir. Also, inhalation of the turpentine oil may produce some hallucinogenic symptoms and hence may be abused leading to toxicity.

Pathophysiology

Turpentine is local irritant. On ingestion, it is rapidly absorbed in the oral cavity and is metabolized by the cytochrome P450 into its metabolites. These conjugated metabolites are excreted through the kidneys.

Symptoms

Symptoms that occur almost immediately after ingestion are:

- Burning sensation in the throat, lips or tongue
- Severe burning sensation along the esophagus
- Pain in abdomen
- Vomiting and nausea
- Difficulty in breathing
- Choking sensation
- Skin irritation and burns
- Hematuria
- Altered mental status
- Convulsions.

Signs

The signs of turpentine toxicity are as follows:

- Hematemesis
- Hematuria
- Severe abdominal pain
- Hypotension
- Tachypnea, tachycardia
- Cyanosis
- Visual disturbances
- Altered sensorium
- Convulsions
- Collapse.

Investigations

1. Routine blood counts may show increased WBC counts, platelet counts may be decreased in turpentine poisoning.
2. Blood levels of turpentine may not be absolutely essential.
3. Chest X-ray: look for evidence of pneumonitis. Usually in asymptomatic patients the X-ray is normal, but signs may develop several hours later.
4. Computed tomography (CT) scan or magnetic resonance imaging (MRI): to be done in case of symptomatic patients to rule out other causes of central nervous system (CNS) symptoms.

Treatment

1. Do not induce emesis, as it increases the likelihood of aspiration.
2. Supportive treatment is indicated.
3. Maintain the airway patency.
4. Administer intravenous (IV) fluids in case of hypotension and ingestion of large quantities of turpentine.

In case of seizures, administer benzodiazepines:

1. Lorazepam is a short-acting antiseizure drug. It acts by increasing the levels of GABA and thus depresses all the

levels of the CNS including the reticular formation and the limbic system.

2. Diazepam also has a short duration of anticonvulsive effect. However, cumulative effects of the drug may occur. It acts by depressing all levels of the CNS.
3. Midazolam is usually used in refractory seizures or in status epilepticus. It has greater affinity to the benzodiazepine receptors in the CNS and takes 2–3 times longer to act than diazepam. Hence, it is recommended to wait for a few more minutes, before repeating the drug dose. Can be administered IM, in case IV access is unavailable.

In case of pneumonitis, the patient needs to be followed up for development and deterioration of the respiratory symptoms. Administer antibiotics, if the possibility of secondary infection exists.

Prognosis

- Usually good
- In case of aspiration pneumonitis, the patient needs to be followed up for further later complications
- Mortality is rare, if early treatment has been administered
- Follow-up counseling and care is essential.

SUGGESTED READING

Kerosene Oil

1. Akamaguna AI, Odita JC. Radiology of kerosene poisoning in young children. Ann Trop Paediatr. 1983;3(2):85-88.
2. Chilcot RP. HPA compendium of chemical hazards: Kerosene (fuel oil) 2007. Version 2. www.hpa.org.uk. Available at www.who.int/ipcs/emergencies/kerosene.pdf [Accessed December, 2012].
3. Goldstein RJ. Hydrocarbons toxicity. www.medscape.com [Accessed April, 2012].
4. Gupta P, Singh RP, Murali MV, et al. Prognostic score for kerosene oil poisoning. Indian Pediatrics. 1992;29(9):1109-112.
5. Health protection agency. Kerosene-Toxicological Review. Available at www.hpa.org.uk/webc/HPAwebFile/HPAweb_C/120 2487083715.
6. Kleigman RM, Behrman RE, Jenson HB, et al. Nelson's Textbook of Pediatrics, 18th edition. Elsevier Health Sciences Division; 2007.

7. Prasad R, Muthusami S, Pandey N, et al. Pneumothorax, subcutaneous emphysema and pneumatocele in a child with accidental kerosene ingestion. Pediatic on call. 2007. www.pediatriconcall.com/fordoctor/viewersChoice/kerosene poisoning.asp [Accessed December, 2012].

Naphthalene

1. American Conference of Governmental Industrial Hygienists (ACGIH). Guide to Occupational Exposure Values. Cincinnati OH; 2003.
2. Delaware Health and Social services: Frequently asked questions on naphthalene poisoning. Information leaflet.
3. Kliegman RM, Behrman RE, Jenson HB, et al. Nelson Textbook of Pediatrics, 18th edition. Elsevier Health Science Division; 2007.
4. Lim HC, Poulose V, Tan HH. Acute naphthalene poisoning following the non-accidental ingestion of mothballs. Singapore Med J. 2009;50(8):e298-301.
5. The US Department of Health and Human Services. Atlanta, GA. Niosh Pocket Guide to Chemical Hazards; 2003.

Turpentine

1. Kashani JS, Tarabar A. Terpene toxicity treatment and management. www.medscape.com [Accessed April, 2011].
2. Kleigman RM, Behrman RE, Jenson HB, et al. Nelson Textbook of Pediatrics, 18th edition. Elsevier Health Sciences Division; 2007.
3. www.nlm.nih.gov/medlineplus/ency/article/002746.htm [Accessed April, 2012].
4. www.osha.gov [Accessed April, 2012].

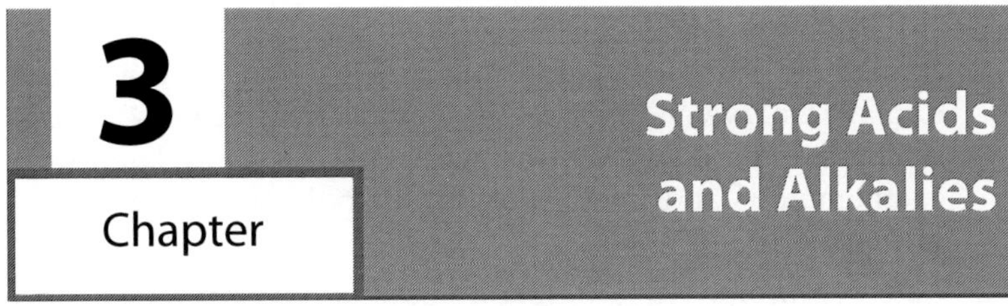

Chapter 3 Strong Acids and Alkalies

PHENOL

ACUTE PHENOL POISONING IN CHILDREN

Phenol poisoning is called carbolism. Phenol is a general protoplasmic poison (denatured protein) with corrosive local effects. Phenol derivates are less toxic than pure phenol. It is also called hydroxybenzene. The lethal dose is from 3 to 30 g, but may be as little as 1 g in children. It causes chemical burns, which could be as severe as burn injury from fire. It has escharotic, as well as neurolytic actions on the human body.

Carbolic acid is a dark brown liquid, which is used as an antiseptic and disinfectant. It is present in cleaning solutions, scouring agents, bleaching agents, oven cleaners and in varying amounts, may be present in soap also.

Due to its easy availability and presence in the home, poisoning with this agent is common in children and adults as well.

Routes

- Accidental oral ingestion
- Surface absorption from skin and wounds
- Serous cavity absorption like from the respiratory tract, due to inhalation of toxic fumes
- Splash injuries to the eyes.

Symptoms

Manifestations of the poisoning depend on the route of absorption of the phenol.

Absorption Through the Skin

1. Immediate symptoms—burning and numbness due to the damaged nerve endings. Dermal exposure produces lesions, which are initially painless white patches and later turn erythematous and finally brown. Phenol produces mucosal burns and coagulum.
2. Late symptoms—white opaque scar is formed, which falls off after some days and leaves a brown stain.
3. Necrosis and gangrene of the affected tissue may be a later manifestation.
4. Occasionally phenol may be absorbed through the conjunctiva, due to accidental splashing on the face. It could result in irritation, scars and damage to the cornea.

Absorption Through the Gastrointestinal Tract

1. Severe intense burning sensation from the mouth till the stomach.
2. Dysphagia, dysarthria, extremely painful deglutition, pain in abdomen, hoarseness of voice.
3. Respiratory tract—involvement may occur due to aspiration, which may occur, while vomiting. It could result in pulmonary edema, laryngeal edema, bronchopneumonia, etc.
4. Late manifestations are the systemic effects, which occur after absorption of the phenol into the system.

Common symptoms: Headache, giddiness, tinnitus, muscular spasms and collapse, unconsciousness, coma, central nervous system (CNS) depression, especially respiratory center depression could occur.

Late Signs

- Breath has a strong odor
- Dilated or constricted pupils
- Hypothermia—temperature fluctuations can occur
- Stertorous breathing
- Cyanosis
- Rapid, feeble, irregular pulse—occasionally rapid pulse

- Urine high colored: oliguria/albuminuria
- Loss of reflex activity
- Tonic seizures may occur
- Weakness, collapse, loss of consciousness
- Initially colorless urine, on exposure to air may change to green/black color. This is due to the oxidation reaction of the excreted phenol into hydroquinone and pyrocatechol and further changes that take place.

Complications

- Shock
- Metabolic acidosis
- Methemoglobinemia
- Cardiac arrhythmias
- Convulsions
- Renal failure
- Corneal scarring
- Esophageal strictures.

Causes of Death

Early: Respiratory failure
Cardiac failure due to shock.

Late: Hepatic failure
Renal failure.

Treatment

Treatment is mainly supportive. The initial priority in treating poisoned children is the standard ABC (airway, breathing and circulation) resuscitation approach.

1. Assess airway patency by looking, listening and feeling for air movement. If there is no air movement, try to open the airway with simple manoeuvres, such as the jaw thrust or the use of airway adjuncts. Phenol, being a caustic agent, may predispose to airway edema.
2. Assess the adequacy of breathing by observing ventilatory frequency, use of accessory muscles, breath sounds and

oxygen saturations. Reduced respiratory effort may require bag-valve-mask ventilation until a definitive airway can be secured.

3. Assess the circulation in terms of cardiovascular status (heart rate, arterial pressure and capillary refill) and the effect of circulatory inadequacy on other organs (mental state, urine output, skin temperature and color). Hypotension should initially be treated with a 20 mL/kg of crystalloid bolus, If the arterial pressure remains resistant to therapy, adequate filling must be ensured in conjunction with the judicious use of inotropic or vasopressor support.

Decontamination

- Remove all the contaminated clothing and discard
- Wash skin copiously with water or if available, use polyethylene glycol or isopropyl alcohol for at least 30 minutes
- If splashed on eyes, irrigate the eyes with plenty of water
- Do not induce emesis
- Careful gastric lavage to empty the stomach contents may be attempted, using activated charcoal with warm water
- Intravenous fluids, normal saline may help in urinary elimination of the toxin. Sodium bicarbonate may be given to counter the metabolic acidosis.

Enhanced Elimination

1. Sometimes, especially with large quantities of phenol poisoning, acute renal failure may develop.
2. In such cases, charcoal hemoperfusion as dialysis useful. This is also useful in cases of poisoning with large amounts of phenol ranging from 15 to 20 g.
3. The rest of the treatment depends on the symptoms expressed in the patient.

Treatment of Complications

Shock: Rapid infusion of IV fluids, normal saline at the rate of 20 mL/kg in half an hour. Follow-up with maintenance fluids. In case of persistent shock, use of inotropic agents dopamine as infusion at the rate of 20–50 μg/min (0.8–1.6 drops/kg/min) to be administered.

Metabolic acidosis: Sodium bicarbonate 1–2 mEq/kg to be administered intravenously, with monitoring of the blood gases.

Methemoglobinemia: To be treated if over 30% or in case of respiratory distress. Administer methylene blue 1–2 mg/kg of 1% solution slow intravenously.

Arrhythmias: Lidocaine in the dose of 1 mg/kg IV as a loading dose. Can be repeated every 5 minutes for a maximum of 3 doses, with electrocardiogram (ECG) monitoring, until reversal of the arrhythmia occurs.

Convulsions: Administer diazepam 0.2–0.3 mg/kg slow IV with ECG monitoring, until the seizure is controlled. Alternatively diazepam may be given rectally for seizure control. In case of refractory seizures, sedation, intubation and ventilation with continuous EEG monitoring will be required.

Renal failure: Forced elimination of the toxin, using charcoal hemoperfusion is indicated.

Corneal scarring: This is usually a late complication. Fluorescein staining and examination of the eye, as soon as the patient stabilizes will be helpful in assessing the extent of corneal damage.

Esophageal strictures: A rare complication in children. May require permanent tracheostomy.

Prognosis

Prognosis of phenol poisoning is usually depends on the amount of toxin exposure and the symptoms expressed by the patient. Complete recovery, without any sequelae may occur.

METHANOL

METHANOL TOXICITY IN CHILDREN

Methanol is also known as 'wood alcohol'. It is used as an industrial solvent. Being a hydrocarbon derivative, it has an aromatic smell, which draws children towards it and hence may be consumed mistakenly by smaller children. Methanol is found commonly in antifreeze, perfumes, paint solvents, photocopying fluid and windshield washing fluid, all of which are readily available.

It is a cheaper derivative than ethanol, which is the constituent of commercially available alcohol. Hence, it is consumed as a cheaper substitute for alcohol and may also be used to adulterate alcohol. Methanol toxicity remains a problem in the lower socioeconomic classes, in many parts of the developing world.

Pathophysiology

Following ingestion, methanol is quickly absorbed into the gastrointestinal tract (GIT) and is metabolized in the liver (Fig. 3.1).

The metabolism of formic acid is very slow, hence following ingestion, there is accumulation of formic acid in the body. Formic acid is known to cause neuronal demyelination. The retrolaminar area of the optic nerve is commonly involved, with intra-axonal swelling, hyperemia, edema, organelle damage and destruction. Optic nerve atrophy can occur. This results in vision loss, which can be one of the early manifestations of methanol toxicity.

The putamen and basal ganglia area of the brain are also affected by methanol toxicity. Hemorrhagic and non-hemorrhagic changes in the putamen are noted, which results in dystonic and parkinsonism like movements. This may be due to the predilection of the striatal neurons to the toxic metabolites of methanol.

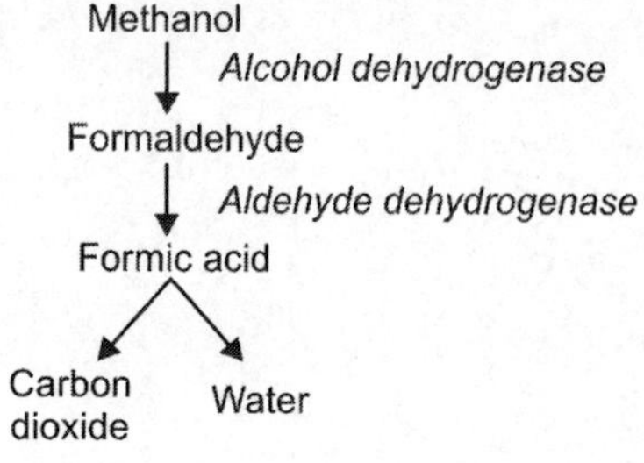

Fig. 3.1: Metabolism of methanol

Hemorrhagic changes are also found in the pancreas and gives rise to symptoms of acute pancreatitis.

Toxic dose: 1 mg/kg has been noted as the minimum lethal dose (MLD) in adults. There is no data of the MLD in children.

Symptoms

The appearance of symptoms depends on the amount of methanol that has been consumed. Usually symptoms appear from 12 to 24 hours after consumption. In case of congestion of ethanol, there may be delay in the appearance of symptoms due to the competitive inhibition that exists between the two compounds. The blood levels of methanol appear to peak from ½ to 1½ after ingestion, hence it essentially does not correlate with the appearance of symptoms.

Central Nervous System

Disinhibition, ataxia, followed by headache, nausea, vomiting and epigastric pain. This could rapidly progress to drowsiness, obtundation and coma. Seizures may manifest later.

Vision Disturbances

Symptoms like blurring of vision, flashing lights and diminished visual acuity. Sometimes, the patient may present with total loss of vision.

Signs

1. Patient seems to be inebriated with ataxia and loss of inhibition.
2. Tachycardia, tachypnea, hypertension and altered mental status could be indicative of ensuing metabolic acidosis.
3. Visual examination shows hyperemia of the optic fundus, which is an early sign. Pupillary light response is compromised and subsequently lost. Scotomata and scintillations may be observed. Blindness occurs due to the accumulation of formic acid in the optic nerve.
4. Pulmonary edema and acute respiratory distress may occur.
5. Hemorrhagic pancreatitis may occur sometimes.
6. Metabolic acidosis develops and is manifested by low serum bicarbonate levels and increased anion gap.

7. Large ingestion of methanol causes depressed myocardial contractility, which could indicate the occurrence of circulatory collapse with cardiac arrhythmias, heart failure or both occurring.

Investigations

1. Serum osmolality: Elevated osmolar gap, which occurs due to the presence of the low molecular weight solutes, like methanol, ethanol, mannitol, proteins, lipids, glycine, etc. Calculate the osmolality using the following formula:

   $$[(\text{mOsm/kg}) = 2\ (\text{Na}^+) + (\text{glucose}/18) + (\text{BUN}/2.8)]$$

2. Serum amylase: Levels are elevated in case of associated hemorrhagic pancreatitis.
3. Serum bicarbonate: Levels are decreased due to the metabolic acidosis. High lactate and ketone levels secondary to formic acid accumulation widen the anion gap.
4. Serum methanol: Levels elevated are a definitive indicator of methanol toxicity. However it is not a good prognostic indicator, as levels rise before the patient is symptomatic.
5. ECG in all leads: In cases of suspected cardiac arrhythmias and to monitor metabolic derangements that can affect cardiac function.
6. USG abdomen: In case of elevated serum amylase, it will show evidence of hemorrhagic pancreatitis that may occur.
7. CT scan brain: May show evidence of putamen necrosis bilaterally with varying degrees of hemorrhage. Cerebral white matter may also show evidence of necrosis.
8. MRI scan of the brain: Localized necrotic lesions of the putamen with or without hemorrhage due to direct toxicity of the methanol metabolites can be seen. Also other cerebral lesions like diffuse cerebral edema, cerebellar necrosis, subcortical white matter necrosis, optic nerve necrosis and intraventricular hemorrhage may be noticed. MRI can be used as a prognosticator and also to differentiate other conditions that may mimic methanol toxicity like carbon monoxide poisoning and hypoglycemia.

Treatment

1. Immediate supportive care: Maintain the airway, provide supplemental oxygen, ensuring adequate breathing and circulation are maintained.
2. Provide adequate hydration to correct the electrolyte imbalance.
3. Administer sodium bicarbonate, which can help to reverse the visual deficits by decreasing the amount of formic acid.
4. Assess the respiration. In case of severe metabolic acidosis, it may be essential to provide assisted ventilation support.
5. In case of seizures, administer anticonvulsants to abort the seizures.
6. Administer antidote therapy: The antidote helps to delay the methanol metabolism until the metabolite is removed from the circulation either naturally or by dialysis.
   a. Ethanol is an antidote for the methanol that has been ingested. It acts by competing with the enzyme alcohol dehydrogenase (ADH), which degrades the methanol to the toxic products. Ethanol has 10–20 times more affinity to the enzyme than methanol and so effectively prevents the formation of formic acid. By elevating the ethanol to reach 100 mg/dL, it acts as a competitive substrate for ADH and is sufficient to block the metabolism of methanol.
   b. Fomepizole is another agent, which acts as a competitive inhibitor to the enzyme ADH, thus reducing the metabolism of methanol. It does not cause sedation or hypoglycemia and is relatively easier to monitor.
7. Hemodialysis: To remove the toxic metabolites and formic acid that has been formed in the body.

   Indications for hemodialysis:

   a. Volume of methanol ingested is more than 30 mL.
   b. Serum methanol level is more than 20 mg/dL.
   c. Visual complications observed.
   d. No improvement in patient's condition and acidosis despite repeated infusion of sodium bicarbonate.

8. Assisted ventilation after intubation; in case the patient has altered sensorium and evidence of respiratory insufficiency, impending cardiac failure, etc.

Prognosis

The prognosis of methanol toxicity depends on the amount of methanol that has been ingested and the time of presentation for treatment.

Indicators of prognosis

1. Large volume of methanol ingested is more than 30 mL.
2. Serum methanol is more than 20 mg/dL.
3. Ocular signs and vision changes.
4. Persistent acidosis.
5. Delayed presentation for treatment.
6. Intractable seizures.
7. Altered sensorium.

ETHYLENE GLYCOL

ETHYLENE GLYCOL POISONING IN CHILDREN

Ethylene glycol belongs to the group of aromatic hydrocarbons and is a toxic alcohol. It is a toxic compound, which is usually a component of the radiator fluids, used in motor vehicles. It is used to increase the boiling point and decrease the freezing point of the fluid that is in circulation inside the vehicle radiator. As it has both the actions, the ethylene glycol can either increase or decrease the fluid temperature, depending on the external weather conditions. Ethylene glycol is also present in solvent as carpet and fabric cleaners.

Ethylene glycol has a characteristic odor and a sweet taste. Hence, it is consumed accidentally often not only by humans, but also by animals.

Pathophysiology

The parent compound, ethylene glycol is non-toxic. It exerts its toxicity after conversion to the active metabolite. It is converted by the enzyme alcohol dehydrogenase to form glycoaldehyde. This enzyme is present in the liver and gastric mucosa. The enzyme aldehdye dehydrogenase then converts the glycoaldehyde into glycolic acid. The toxic features of ethylene glycol are attributed to the presence of glycolic acid, which provides an acidic milieu, thus stimulating acidosis. This glycolate is then transformed into glyoxylic acid, which could then be transformed into the highly toxic oxalate or the safer glutamate or α-ketoadipic acid metabolites. The oxalate crystals enter the urine, where they precipitate with calcium to form calcium oxalate crystals, which accumulate in the renal cortex, tissues and blood. The renal flow is decreased, glomerular filtration rate (GFR) reduces and renal insufficiency results. Since calcium is drawn from the circulation, its level in the blood falls resulting in hypocalcemia (Fig. 3.2).

Toxic dose: Approximately, 1.0–1.5 mL/kg or 100 mL in an adult.

Symptoms

The clinical syndrome of ethylene glycol intoxication has traditionally been divided into three stages as given below:

1. Progressive involvement of the CNS.
2. Involvement of cardiopulmonary systems.

3. Involvement of the kidneys.
    - Symptoms usually non-specific
    - Nausea, vomiting
    - Heavy deep breathing
    - Seizures
    - Altered sensorium.

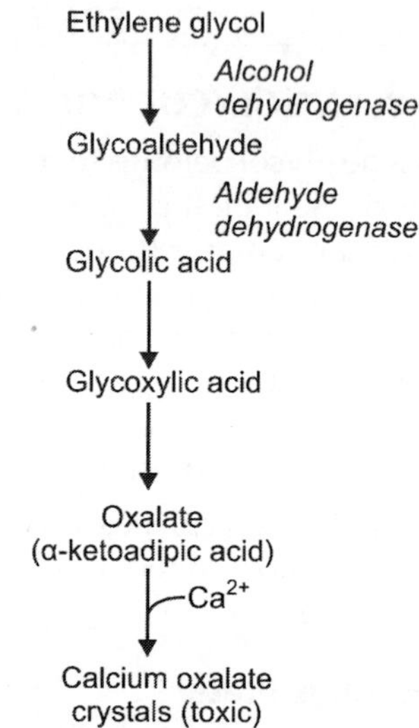

Fig. 3.2: Pathophysiology of ethylene glycol poisoning

Signs

- Rapid deep breathing
- Kussmaul breathing
- Dehydration due to persistent vomiting
- Muscle tetany due to hypocalcemia
- Hypertension
- Cardiac failure
- Seizures.

Investigations

1. Routine blood counts.
2. Serum electrolytes—calcium, sodium, potassium, bicarbonate can reveal anion gap, metabolic acidosis.
3. Blood glucose levels—to rule out diabetic ketoacidosis.
4. Arterial blood gases—ion gap estimation.
5. Measurement of serum osmolality—is done by measuring a set of electrolytes, sodium, BUN, glucose levels. The observed osmolality is calculated using a formula:
    - 2 × Na + level + BUN level/3 + glucose level/18

    The serum osmolality is then calculated using the freezing point technique. The difference between the serum osmolality and the calculated osmolality is equal to the osmolality gap. Once the osmolality gap is obtained, the serum levels of ethylene glycol can be obtained by multiplying with the conversion factor of 6.2.

6. Colorimetric tests to determine serum levels of ethylene glycol—currently this test is not widely available at many centers.
7. Urine exam—shows the presence of calcium oxalate crystals. This is a late sign of toxicity. Calcium oxalate crystals appear in many forms, the most common being is needle-shaped monohydrate. The characteristic appearance like a folded envelope of the oxalate crystals are seen later and with high concentration only.
8. Wood's lamp examination of urine—on shining the Wood's lamp, if the urine has ethylene glycol, it will give a greenish colored glow in a dark room. This is due to the presence of fluorescein in the radiator fluid.
9. ECG in all leads—for the possibility of any cardiac abnormalities, arrhythmias due to associated electrolyte abnormalities.
10. CT scan of the brain—to rule out any associated CNS causes of altered sensorium.

Treatment

1. Stabilize the airway.
2. Ensure the breathing is maintained. Administer supplemental oxygen.
3. Insert the IV cannula to maintain the circulation and adequate volume correction.
4. Administer IV crystalloids rapidly, to enhance the renal elimination of the toxin and to prevent its deposition in the renal cortices. It has to be administered rapidly, as much as 250–500 mL/h, which will also help to maintain the blood pressure of the patient.
5. Catheterize the patient, especially with altered sensorium. This will help to estimate the urine output, measure serially for the presence of oxalate crystals and give an idea of the renal clearance of the toxin.
6. In case of acidosis, administer sodium bicarbonate IV, diluted 1–2 mEq/kg slowly.
7. As pyridoxine and thiamine act as cofactors in the metabolism of ethylene glycol, they may be administered parenterally to aid the elimination of the toxin. Pyridoxine enhances

the conversion of glyoxylate to glycine. Thiamine catalyzes the conversion of glycolic acid to glyoxylate and its further conversion to a non-toxic metabolite, alpha-hydroxy-beta-ketoadipate.

8. In case of evidence of hypocalcemia, administer calcium slowly by IV.

Antidote

The specific antidote for ethylene glycol is fomepizole [4-methylpyrazole (4MP), Antizol]. This is the specific antidote, which does not depress the CNS, causes no respiratory depression, no hypoglycemia and is safe to use. It acts competitively to inhibit the formation of the toxic aldehyde and the glyoxylic acid in the blood. Fomepizole treatment should be initiated as soon as possible when ethylene glycol poisoning is suspected. Inhibition of metabolite production begins within 3 hours of initiating therapy with fomepizole and resolution of acidosis occurs, the anion gap is normalized within 4 hours. If fomepizole therapy is begun before a rise in the serum creatinine concentration, damage to the kidney can be avoided.

Indications for antidote therapy:

1. Ethylene glycol levels in plasma more than 20 mg/dL.
2. Definite history of recent ingestion of ethylene glycol.
3. Osmolal gap more than 10 mOsm/L.
4. Suspected ingestion of ethylene glycol associated with at least two of the following:
   - Osmolal gap more than 10 mOsm/L
   - Serum bicarbonate less than 20 mEq/L
   - Arterial pH more than 7.3
   - Presence of urine oxalate crystals.

Fomepizole needs to be administered parenterally, slow IV over 30 minutes. Start as a loading dose, usually 15 mg/kg followed by repeat doses at 12 hour intervals calculated at 10 mg/kg for four doses. After this, continued dosing needs to be done at 15 mg/kg/12 hours. It can also be administered orally, in case the ICU setting is not available. However, it is an expensive drug and not easily available.

In the absence of fomepizole, ethanol can be used as an antidote. It acts by saturating the enzyme alcohol dehydrogenase. It can be given orally or parenterally. The recommended dose for IV ethanol is given as a 10% solution, diluted in 5% dextrose. The loading dose is 8–10 mL/kg given over a 30 minute period, followed by the maintenance dose of 1.4–2 mL/kg/h. Intravenous administration of ethanol should be continued until ethylene glycol levels have been reduced below 20 mg/dL and the metabolic acidosis has been corrected. The aim is to maintain serum levels above 100 mg/dL. Careful monitoring of the levels are needed to avoid over medication with ethanol. However, the treatment with ethanol has disadvantages, due to its variable metabolism, CNS depression and difficulty in maintaining effective serum concentrations.

Hemodialysis

Hemodialysis is essential to remove the toxic metabolites in case the patient has presented with metabolic acidosis.

Indications for hemodialysis:

- Late presentation
- Severe metabolic acidosis
- Acute renal failure
- Anuria
- Severe renal dysfunction despite treatment with antidotes.

Prolonged dialysis may not be necessary in patients treated with fomepizole or ethanol. Serum osmolality levels and electrolyte levels should be monitored closely every 2–4 hours for 12–24 hours following the discontinuation of dialysis because redistribution of ethylene glycol may result in an elevated serum concentration. Hemodialysis is essential to promote the conversion of intermediate byproducts into non-toxic metabolites. The end point for dialysis in these patients is correction of the anion and osmolar gaps. Ongoing administration of calcium may be essential to combat associated hypocalcemic tetany.

Pyridoxine and thiamine may be administered to accelerate the conversion of the intermediate products to non-toxic end products. The thiamine may also be indicated in case symptoms of ethanol withdrawal are suspected.

Peritoneal dialysis is not useful, as the ethylene glycol anions cannot be cleared adequately by this route.

Prognosis

In case of early adequate treatment of the toxicity, the patient usually recovers completely.

Causes of Death

- Severe metabolic acidosis
- Uncontrolled seizures
- Renal failure.

SUGGESTED READING

Phenol

1. Allen R. Chemical safety data sheets. Vol 4b: toxic chemicals (m-z). Royal Society of Chemistry, Cambridge. 1991.
2. Kleigman RM, Behrman RE, Jenson HB, et al. Nelson Textbook of Pediatrics, 18th edition. Elsevier Health Sciences Division; 2007.
3. Phenol: International Program on Chemical Safety. Poisons Information Monograph 412, Chemical.

Methanol

1. Kleigman RM, Behrman RE, Jenson HB, et al. Nelson Textbook of Pediatrics, 18th edition. Elsevier Health Sciences Division; 2007.
2. Korabathina K. Methanol toxicity. www.medscape.com [Accessed May, 2012].

Ethylene Glycol

1. Keyes DC, Tarabar A. Toxicity: Ethylene glycol. www.medscape.com [Accessed May, 2012].
2. Kleigman RM, Behrman RE, Jenson HB, et al. Nelson Textbook of Pediatrics, 18th edition. Elsevier Health sciences Division; 2007.
3. Kraut AJ, Kurtz I. Toxic alcohol ingestions: Clinical features, diagnosis and management. Clin J Am Soc Nephrol. 2008;3(1):208-25.
4. Scalley RD, Ferguson DR, Piccaro JC, et al. Treatment of ethylene glycol poisoning. Am Fam Physician. 2002;66(5):807-12.

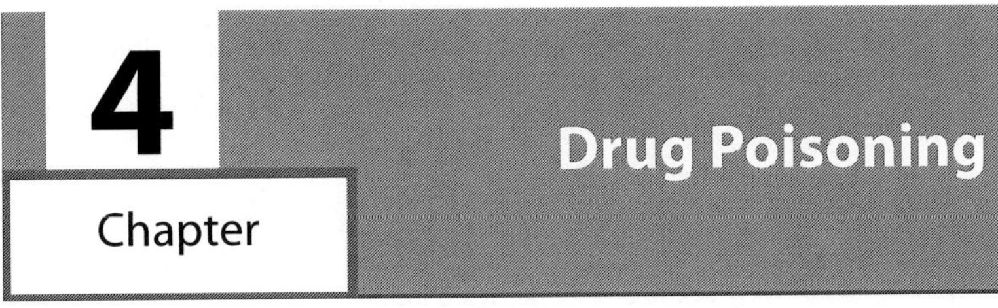

Chapter 4 Drug Poisoning

PARACETAMOL

ACETAMINOPHEN/PARACETAMOL POISONING

Paracetamol is frequently used as an antipyretic analgesic drug in children. It is easily available as an over-the-counter (OTC) medication. Since the contraindication to the use of Aspirin was widely made known, paracetamol or acetaminophen has been widely used, especially in children.

Paracetamol is available as a single agent drug or in combination with other pharmaceutical agents, in various formulations. The chemical formulation is N-acetyl-p-aminophenol (APAP), which is generally a safe drug when used in the correct therapeutic dosage.

Toxic dose: More than 150–200 mg/kg as a single acute ingestion.

Pathophysiology

Upon ingestion, paracetamol is rapidly absorbed by the gastrointestinal tract (GIT) and peak serum levels of the drug occur after 0.5–2 hours, after ingestion. The metabolism of the drug is essentially hepatic and the liver metabolizes over 90% of the drug to the water-soluble compounds of sulfate and glucuronide. While sulfation is the predominant pathway of metabolism in the younger children, glucuronide formation occurs in children over 12 years and the conjugates are easily excreted in the urine due to water solubility.

N-acetyl-p-benzoquinone imine (NAPQI) is the toxic metabolite, which cannot be detoxified by the body. It binds to the hepatocytes at the lipid bilayer and causes centrilobular necrosis. Metabolism of paracetamol is given in Figure 4.1.

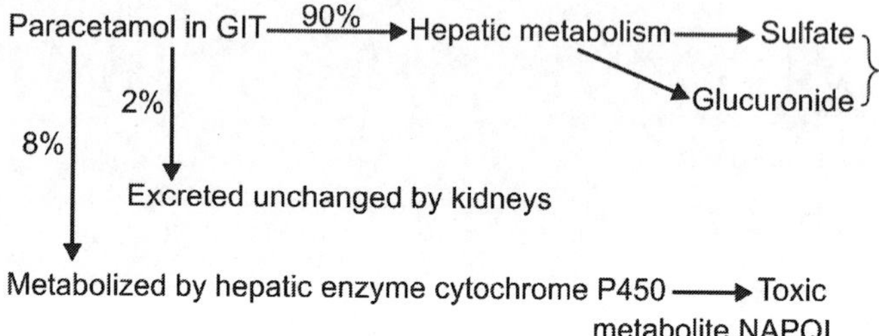

Fig. 4.1: Metabolism of paracetamol

The therapeutic levels of paracetamol are 10–20 μg/mL. The elimination half-life is 2–4 hours. Coingestion with drugs, which delay the gastric emptying like anticholinergics, opiates, etc. as well as use of the extended release products will delay the elimination and increase the peak serum levels. Glutathione binds to the toxic metabolite NAPQI forming the non-toxic mercapturate conjugate, which is excreted by the urine.

Therapeutic dose in children: 10–15 mg/kg/dose every 4–6 hourly.

The single dose that can result in toxicity is higher in the younger children between 1 and 6 years, due to the higher hepatic mass in this age group, which effectively detoxifies even larger doses of ingested acetaminophen.

Toxic Dose

- 150–200 mg/dose—toxic
- 250 mg/dose—significant hepatotoxicity
- More than 350 mg/dose—severe hepatotoxicity.

Signs and Symptoms

Acetaminophen toxicity presents in four clinical stages depending on the period of presentation after ingestion.

Stage I

1. Lasts for the initial 24 hours.
2. Patient may be asymptomatic.
3. Patients present with nausea, vomiting, malaise. Non-specific signs, hence the patient may receive additional doses of paracetamol as treatment.

4. In case, there is severe metabolic acidosis or neurologic signs noted, consider the possibility of coingestants.
5. Signs are non-specific and include pallor, diaphoresis and altered hydration status due to the recurrent vomiting and insensible fluid loss.
6. Blood parameters are within normal limits. However, post-ingestion after 12 hours, there may be some alteration in the hepatic enzyme levels, especially aspartate aminotransferase (AST) and alanine aminotransferase (ALT).

Stage II

1. Lasts from 24 to 48 hours postingestion.
2. Pain in the right upper quadrant of the abdomen along with decreased urine output may be noted.
3. Tenderness in the right upper quadrant, with hepatomegaly is noted. Acute pancreatitis may coexist occasionally in children, but is common in alcoholics.
4. Serum levels of AST, ALT, prothrombin time (PT) and bilirubin levels are elevated, while renal function tests are also impaired.

Stage III

1. Lasts from 3 to 5 days after ingestion.
2. Stage I symptoms, along with signs of hepatic failure appear.
3. Jaundice, coagulopathy, hypoglycemia, encephalopathy and/or sepsis occur. Renal failure along with cardiomyopathy may occur.
4. Jaundice, abdominal pain, GIT bleeds point towards hepatotoxicity. Cerebral edema and encephalopathy may occur with severe liver damage. In case of large amounts ingested and in some cases with toxic doses, there could be evidence of fulminant hepatic failure and multiorgan failure.
5. Laboratory investigations shows the evidence of severe hepatotoxicity. Marked elevations in AST greater than 10,000, ALT, prolonged PT and international normalized ratio (INR), serum bilirubin above 4 mg/dL, lactic acidosis and hyperammonemia are noted. Renal function tests show abnormal results with proteinuria, hematuria and granular

casts. Renal failure is usually associated with over 50% of hepatic failure patients.

6. Liver biopsy reveals centrilobular necrosis, which could progress to acute fulminant hepatic failure.
7. Multiorgan failure is usually the cause of death in this stage.

Stage IV

1. Lasts from 5 to 14 days up to 3 weeks after ingestion of toxic doses.
2. This could be the stage of recovery or the stage of death. The clinical recovery occurs faster than the cytological recovery, which normally takes several weeks.

There could be some residual abnormality in hepatic function after toxic dose ingestion.

Risk Factors for Paracetamol Toxicity

1. Malnourished children.
2. Prolonged fasting.
3. Gastroenteritis.
4. HIV infection.
5. Coadministration of hepatotoxic medications like INH, rifampicin, phenytoin, phenobarbital, trimethoprim sulfamethoxazole, etc.
6. Some herbal health supplements.

The risk factors act by depleting the body glutathione levels. The drugs act by activating the cytochrome P450 system, which increases the levels of NAPQI in the body and hence, aggravates the paracetamol-induced hepatotoxicity.

Chronic Paracetamol Toxicity

Chronic paracetamol toxicity occurs in young children who are unwell and who receive repeated doses of paracetamol, along with poor oral intake. The glutathione stores may be reduced as well as the metabolism could be increased in these children, which together contributes to the chronic toxicity. Diagnosis is difficult as the initial symptoms may mimic the acute febrile illness.

Maintain maximum daily dose of paracetamol below 80 mg/kg /day to prevent occurrence of toxicity.

Investigations

1. Routine blood counts—will show evidence of coexistent infection.
2. Liver function tests—extent of liver damage can be approximated. Transaminase levels begin to rise by 24 hours and peak between 48 and 72 hours after ingestion. In sever toxicity, elevated levels will be noted within 12–16 hours.
3. Serum glucose levels—to rule out hyperglycemia.
4. Coagulation profile—disturbed in gross liver damage.
5. Serum ammonia level—in case of altered mental status, will give information regarding coexistent encephalopathy.
6. Renal function tests—to detect renal failure, which can occur independent of liver failure. Usually becomes apparent in stage II after ingestion.
7. Routine urinalysis—can help to detect the acute tubular necrosis.
8. Serum acetaminophen level, salicylate level—to detect coingestants.
9. Ultrasonography (USG) abdomen—will show disturbances in liver and/or renal pathology.
10. Liver biopsy—changes could range from hepatic cytolysis to centrilobular necrosis. Occurrence of centrilobular damage could point towards fulminant hepatic failure.
11. CT scan of the head—in case of altered mental status, encephalopathy or suspected cerebral edema.
12. Rumack-Matthew nomogram—is used to interpret and assess the possibility of hepatotoxicity in patients with paracetamol overdose. It is useful as a one time predictor of outcome, but cannot be used to estimate the future possibility or risk of fulminant hepatic failure in the patient. Nomogram tracking can begin as early as 4 hours after ingestion and is valid until 24 hours after ingestion.

Treatment

1. Supportive care—maintain the airway, breathing and circulation.
2. Adequate hydration—administer intravenous (IV) fluids.
3. GIT decontamination—use activated charcoal, in case patient presents within 4 hours after ingestion. Airway protection is essential before decontamination.

Activated charcoal acts by preventing the absorption of the drug by the intestine. The charcoal adsorbs the drug, decreases its enterohepatic recirculation and increases the enterocapillary reabsorption. Best results are obtained, if it is administered within 30 minutes of drug ingestion.

Dose

- Infants: 1 g/kg/dose, may be repeated after 4–6 hours
- Children: 1–2 g/kg/dose orally, may be repeated after 4–6 hours.

Contraindications to Activated Charcoal

1. Intestinal obstruction.
2. Unprotected airway.
3. Caustic ingestion: In case patient is seen early, within 1 hour after ingestion gastric lavage may be performed.
4. Specific antidote: The specific antidote for acetaminophen poisoning is N-acetylcysteine (NAC), which can be given orally or by intravenous administration.

N-ACETYLCYSTEINE

N-acetylcysteine acts by replenishment of the glutathione stores, which helps to decrease paracetamol/acetaminophen toxicity. It also directly detoxifies the NAPQI to produce the non-toxic metabolites, which are then excreted. It also provides a substrate for sulfation, which increase the non-toxic metabolite produced; besides, it causes direct conjugation of the NAPQI, which further reduces the toxicity of the drug in the body.

For best results, the antidote needs to be administered within 8–10 hours of acetaminophen ingestion.

Indications for Use of IV NAC

1. Altered mental status.
2. Severe toxicity.
3. GIT bleeding.
4. GIT obstruction.
5. History of caustic ingestion.
6. Refractory emesis despite adequate antiemetics.

Method of Administration

N-acetylcysteine is available as a 20% solution (200 mg/mL). This needs to be diluted to a 5% solution, i.e. 50 mg/mL by using fruit juice or a carbonated beverage.

If the patient vomits within 60 minutes of administration, repeat the entire dose. If it is to be given IV, the formulation is diluted using 5% dextrose in water and infused .

Aggressive antiemetics need to be administered in case the patient vomits due to associated nausea or due to smell of the NAC. It is preferable to use antiemetics, which do not decrease the gastric motility, hence avoid the use of anticholinergic antiemetics like prochlorperazine and phenothiazines, which may actually worsen the symptoms of toxicity.

Protocols for Administration of NAC

- < 2 hours—oral administration
- 21 hours—intravenous administration
- 48 hours—intravenous administration.

Delayed presentation of acute single ingestion of paracetamol: Current recommendations suggest use of NAC for patients who present over 24 hours after ingestion, if there is evidence of hepatotoxicity and if there is unmetabolized acetaminophen detected in the serum. Laboratory evidence of disordered liver function test (LFT) is an indication for use of NAC. Treatment can be continued based on the clinical improvement noted.

Liver Transplantation

Liver transplantation is indicated in patients, who suffer from severe liver damage and may provide a possibility of liver recovery.

Indications for Liver Transplantation: King's College Criteria

1. pH less than 7.30 after fluid resuscitation.
2. Serum creatinine more than 3.3 mg/dL.
3. PT more than 1.8 time control or PT more than 100 seconds or INR more than 6.5.
4. Grade III or higher encephalopathy.

Prognosis

In cases of acute exposure, the morbidity and mortality rates are lower in children less than 5 years than the older children and adolescents, probably due to better glutathione stores and increased capacity to conjugation and greater likelihood to vomit after ingestion.

Indicators of Poor Prognosis

1. Grade III or higher encephalopathy.
2. PT more than 1.8 times control levels.
3. INR more than 6.5.
4. Serum creatinine more than 3.3 mg/dL.
5. Serum phosphate more than 1.2 mmol/L at 48–96 hours after overdose.
6. Blood lactate more than 3.5 mmol/L before fluid resuscitation or more than 3 mmol/L after adequate fluid resuscitation.

NON-STEROIDAL ANTI-INFLAMMATORY DRUGS

NON-STEROIDAL ANTI-INFLAMMATORY POISONING IN CHILDREN

Non-steroidal anti-inflammatory drugs (NSAIDs) are used as antipyretics, anti-inflammatory agents, painkillers and in the treatment of juvenile rheumatoid arthritis. Poisoning with these drugs may occur due to accidental overdosage or may occasionally be intentional.

Pathophysiology

Cyclooxygenase (COX) is an enzyme that catalyzes the conversion of arachidonic acid to prostaglandins and thromboxane. This enzyme is reversibly inhibited by NSAIDs, resulting in decreased pain and inflammation. The COX enzyme is present as two forms: COX-1 and COX-2. The COX-1 is present in all the tissues and is associated with production of prostaglandins that protect the gastric mucosa, maintain organ function and produce thromboxane, which is essential for platelet aggregation and vasoconstriction. COX-2 is associated with prostaglandins that are associated with inflammation and pain and are also expressed on the kidneys and vascular endothelium. NSAIDs are thus useful in decreasing pain and inflammation. The prostaglandins are thus involved in maintaining the gastric mucosal integrity and also the renal blood flow and vasoconstriction. The older NSAIDs are COX-1 inhibitors, while the newer ones are selective COX-2 inhibitors, thus decreasing the gastric side effects. However in case of overdosage, the selectivity of the drugs is lost.

Drug Interactions

The toxicity of the NSAIDs is aggravated by the coadministration of other drugs along with it. Aminoglycosides, phenytoin, digoxin, lithium, oral hypoglycemics are some of the drugs that interact and aggravate the toxicity of NSAIDs. Acetaminophen is usually coadministered with NSAIDs and may aggravate the toxicity of the NSAID.

NSAIDs are available in different classes:

- Pyrazolones, e.g. phenylbutazone, a potently toxic NSAID
- Fenamates, e.g. mefenamic acid

- Acetic acids, e.g. diclofenac, indomethacin, sulindac
- COX-2 inhibitors, e.g. celecoxib, which is relatively safe
- Propionic acid, e.g. ibuprofen, naproxen, ketoprofen
- Oxicams, e.g. piroxicam.

All NSAIDs can produce toxic symptoms. However, the most severe effects have been found to occur following overdose of mefenamic acid, phenylbutazone and meclofenamate sodium containing preparations.

Symptoms

- Nausea and vomiting
- Dyspepsia
- Abdominal pain
- Drowsiness and lethargy
- Ataxia
- Nystagmus
- Altered sensorium
- Coma
- Tinnitus and hearing loss
- Refractory acidosis
- Multiorgan failure.

Signs

- Tachypnea, bradypnea
- Acidosis—early respiratory or metabolic
- Hypertension—due to fluid retention, antagonistic action of NSAIDs on beta blockers, angiotensin-converting enzyme (ACE) inhibitors and diuretics
- Gallop rhythm, S3 may be heard
- Occasionally, dysrhythmias may occur in worsening heart failure
- Angioedema, flushing, rhinorrhea
- Pain abdomen, signs of gastrointestinal (GI) bleeding
- Wheezing

- Respiratory arrest
- Myoclonus
- Seizures.

Late Signs

- Hepatic failure
- Renal failure
- Jaundice
- Platelet dysfunction
- Heart failure
- Metabolic acidosis.

Investigations

1. Complete blood count (CBC), including platelet count.
2. Coagulation studies, including PT and INR.
3. Serum levels of NSAID, Aspirin, acetaminophen.
4. Serum electrolytes, bicarbonate, lactate, magnesium and phosphorus levels, especially in patients with central nervous system (CNS) symptoms.
5. Liver function tests in all patients, which can act as a baseline guide value.
6. Renal function tests especially in cases of overdose with mefenamic acid, phenylbutazone and meclofenamate containing drugs.
7. Serum acetaminophen levels need to be evaluated at 4 hours after ingestion to rule out coingestions, as initial values may be normal.
8. ECG in all leads, to rule out dysrhythmias, as well as to look for evidence of hyperkalemia.
9. Abdominal X-ray: in case of persistent vomiting, if perforation is suspected.
10. Chest X-ray: also indicated in case of suspected viscous perforation.
11. CT scan of the brain: to be done in patient with altered mental status, recurrent seizures or comatose patient.

Treatment

No Specific Antidote for NSAID Toxicity

1. Maintain the airway. Ensure patient is alert and able to maintain the gag reflex, else intubate and ventilate the patient.
2. Administer supplemental oxygen.
3. Insert the IV line and administer IV fluids at maintenance levels, unless sever vomiting occurs, with likelihood of dehydration.
4. Gastric decontamination—to be done after ensuring that the airway is protected and patient is able to maintain the gag reflex, to avoid likelihood of aspiration.

   Activated charcoal is administered if patient presents within 4 hours after ingestion. In case of massive ingestion in the intubated patient, orogastric lavage may be performed to eliminate the ingested drug.
5. In case of acidosis, administer sodium bicarbonate IV.
6. Enhanced elimination.
   a. Hemodialysis is indicated in patients with acute renal failure, severe volume depletion, refractory lactic acidosis, critically ill patient, multisystem failure.
   b. Extracorporeal membrane oxygenation (ECMO)—used to treat massive ibuprofen overdosage.
7. In case of convulsions, administer benzodiazepines to abort the seizures. They tend to be short lived and hence usually do not require repeated medication. However, in case of recurrent seizures, administer barbiturates.
8. Proton pump inhibitors and H2 receptor antagonists may be useful to counter the GIT effects of the NSAIDs. However, their efficacy has not been proven, unless massive GIT bleeds have been detected.

Prognosis

Usually favorable outcome, especially if early treatment has been administered.

BARBITURATES

BARBITURATE POISONING IN CHILDREN

Barbiturates are sedative-hypnotic drugs, that have been used classically for the treatment of epilepsy.

Pathophysiology

Barbiturates are the derivative drugs from barbituric acid. They act by binding to the gamma-aminobutyric acid (GABA) receptors and allow the influx of chloride ions, resulting in hyperpolarization of the postsynaptic neurons. This potentiates and prolongs the action of GABA, which is an inhibitory neurotransmitter in the CNS. Barbiturates also block glutamate, which is an excitatory neurotransmitter.

They are classified into:

1. Long acting: Duration of action over 6 hours.
2. Short acting:
   - Ultrashort-acting duration of action for few minute
   - Short-acting duration of action less than 3 hours
   - Intermediate-acting duration of action from 3 to 6 hours.

Long-acting barbiturates are less lipid soluble than the short acting ones. They accumulate more slowly in the tissues and are readily excreted by the kidneys as the active drug. For example, phenobarbital, primidone, etc.

Short-acting barbiturates are more lipid soluble, more protein bound, have a more rapid onset of action and are metabolized by the liver, e.g. thiopental, secobarbital, etc.

Effects of Barbiturates

Barbiturates have effects mainly on the CNS, besides the pulmonary and cardiovascular side effects (Box 4.1). These effects are mainly depressive and its effects depend on the duration of action and the half-life of the drug ingested. The short-acting barbiturates have a half-life of less than 40 hours, while the long-acting barbiturates have a half-life of over 40 hours and hence cause more prolonged depressive effects.

Central Nervous System Effects

Barbiturates have CNS depressive and sedative effects, due to their effect of hyperpolarization of the cell membranes. Hence, they are useful drugs for treatment of epilepsy. At lower doses, they cause sedation and hypnosis. Some drugs are more lipophilic and hence penetrate the brain tissue rapidly causing anesthesia, which is usually short lived.

Pulmonary Effects

Barbiturates cause medullary respiratory center depression, thus inducing respiratory depression. Hypoxia ensues and is responsible for most of the secondary manifestations of the drug. Fatality is normally secondary to respiratory depression followed by secondary pneumonia.

Cardiovascular System Effects

Medullary vasomotor center depression can cause cardiac depression. At higher doses, it affects the contractility and vascular tone, vasodilatation, resulting in cardiac collapse.

- Toxic dose: More than 300 mg of phenobarbitone
- Lethal dose: Over 1 g of phenobarbitone.

What happens when a toddler ingests over 10 tablets of Gardenal sodium?

1. Almost 100% of the ingested phenobarbitone is absorbed by the body.
2. Maximum levels are achieved after 1–18 hours of ingestion.
3. Rate of absorption varies depending on the dissolution of the particular formulation ingested.
4. Absorbed particles are rapidly distributed to most tissues of the body.
5. Duration of action depends on the hepatic metabolism and renal elimination.

Box 4.1: Shows effects of barbiturates on various systems

Central nervous system
- Sedative-depressive effect

Pulmonary
- Medullary center depression

Cardiovascular system
- Medullary vasomotor center depression

Symptoms

The patients with suspected barbiturate overdose must be thoroughly examined, as he/she can present with a variety of symptoms as mentioned in Table 4.1.

Table 4.1: Common symptoms of barbiturate poisoning

Central nervous system	Cardiovascular system	Respiratory
Lethargy, hypothermia	Tachycardia, bradycardia	Apnea
Ataxia, slurred speech	Hypotension	Hypoxia
Nystagmus, strabismus	Diaphoresis	Respiratory depression
Vertigo	Shock	Acute respiratory distress syndrome
Hypothermia		

Other Manifestations

1. Gastrointestinal tract: Decreased bowel movements.
2. Psychiatric: Impaired thinking, irritability, aggressiveness.
3. Skin: Barbiturate blisters, bullous lesions on knees, buttocks and hands over an erythematous area.

Signs

Signs of barbiturate intoxication depend on the severity of intoxication.

1. Drowsiness—the degree of drowsiness or unconsciousness depends on the amount of intoxication.
2. Decreased papillary reflexes.
3. Tachycardia/bradycardia.
4. Decreased deep tendon reflexes.
5. Hypothermia.
6. Signs of shock.
7. Acute respiratory distress syndrome.
8. Apnea.
9. Decreased bowel sounds.

Laboratory Investigations

1. Complete blood count, serum electrolytes, serum creatinine, blood urea and blood glucose levels will help to rule out altered consciousness due to metabolic derangements.
2. Arterial blood gases—helps to determine the presence of metabolic acidosis, respiratory failure and hypoxia. Also can be used as a baseline measure in case the patient needs to be ventilated.
3. Serum barbiturate levels—helpful if levels can be estimated. Can be used as a guide to prognosis, type of treatment and elimination methods to be utilized, as well as the efficacy of treatment.
   - Levels above 35 mg/dL for short-acting barbiturates, indicates poor prognosis
   - Levels above 90 mg/dL for long-acting barbiturates indicates poor prognosis.
4. ECG—to assess the cardiac status at admission and to monitor the patient for any possible complications. Rhythm disturbances can occur with hypothermia and can result in ventricular fibrillation, if core temperature drops further.

Treatment

Emergency Care

Supportive care is essential in treatment of barbiturate poisoning are as follows:

1. Airway maintenance: Assess the adequacy of the airway and respiration. Administer supplemental oxygen. If altered sensorium, intubate the patient and provide assisted ventilation. Continuous monitoring of the airway status is essential to check for any deterioration in the patient's condition.
2. Check the body temperature, if possible the rectal temperasture to gauge the core temperature. If hypothermic, carefully rewarm the patient, to prevent any further fall on blood pressure due to hypothermia.
3. Administer IV fluids and aggressively treat the hypovolemic shock. If the shock persists despite the aggressive fluid replacement, administer vasopressors, e.g. dopamine, IV (dose: 5–10 μg/kg/min as continuous infusion).

4. Gastric decontamination:
   a. Gastric lavage—to be initiated after patient is hemodynamically stabilized.
   b. Nasogastric tube is inserted.
   c. Activated charcoal is used to adsorb the ingested phenobarbitone.
   d. Dosage: 1 g/kg of activated charcoal is administered initially. Repeated doses of activated charcoal may be required to facilitate the decontamination.
   e. A cathartic is usually administered once charcoal is used, to facilitate the gastric emptying. This is because the barbiturate per se slows down the gastric emptying and decreases the gastric motility.
   f. Induced emesis is contraindicated, due to the risk of aspiration that could occur because of the depressed neurologic status of the patient.
5. Forced alkaline diuresis is used to aid in the expulsion of the barbiturate ions especially in cases of moderate-to-severe poisoning and in cases of long-acting barbiturate toxicity. It is not indicated for short-acting barbiturate toxicity as these are primarily metabolized in the liver. High water solubility, lower hepatic metabolism and longer half-life of the drugs like phenobarbital, butabarbital, etc. make the drug ionized and lipid insoluble, so that they cannot diffuse back to the extracellular fluid, hence get trapped by the alkaline urine and can be excreted. Bladder catheterization may help to measure the urine volume accurately.

To prepare the fluid: Use 0.5 normal saline or 5% dextrose to which, add 50–150 mEq of sodium bicarbonate per liter of the fluid, resulting in an isotonic fluid.

Rate of administration of the fluid: 1–2 L/h for 2–3 hours. After that, titrate the fluid administered to the amount of urine output, usually around 500 mL/h. Add 20–40 mEq/L of KCL, after adequate urine output and in case of hypokalemia during diuresis. Use of a diuretic, like 10% mannitol or furosemide can be added to promote the diuresis. Monitor urine pH. Maintain urine pH between 7.5 and 8.5. Complications and contraindications of alkaline diuresis is shown in Figure 4.2.

6. Extracorporeal elimination of the drug is rarely required. This method includes hemoperfusion and hemodialysis. Hemoperfusion is preferred, as the clearance rates are better than with dialysis.

   Indications for hemoperfusion or hemodialysis:

   a. Severe barbiturate intoxication, serum concentration greater than 100 mg/L.
   b. Severe shock.
   c. Stage IV coma.
   d. Renal failure.
   e. Severe hypothermia.
   f. Pulmonary edema.
   g. Comatose patient with apnea.
   h. Unresponsive to other methods of drug elimination.

Hemoperfusion involves circulating the blood through an extracorporeal circuit, which contains an absorbent like activated charcoal or polystyrene resin. The thin membrane has a larger surface area for the drug adhesion and its subsequent elimination from the blood.

Hemodialysis involves circulation of the blood through an extracorporeal membrane. It is indicated when the endogenous clearance of the drug is low, when the patient's condition is progressively deteriorating or when the drug levels are indicative of a poor outcome.

Peritoneal dialysis is seldom used as the drug clearance is poor. It is indicated only when the other methods of

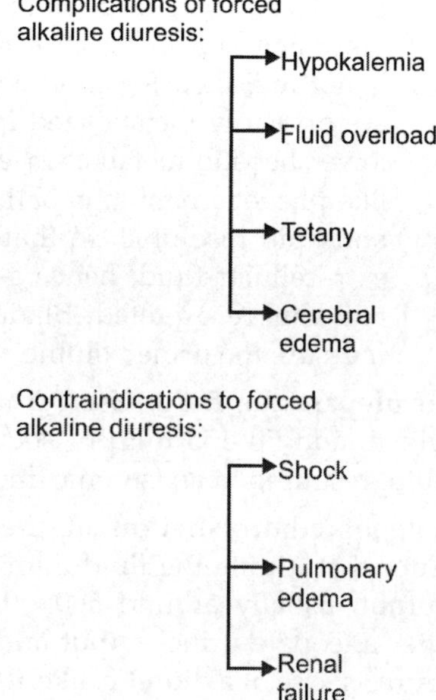

Fig. 4.2: Complication and contraindication of forced alkaline diuresis

extracorporeal clearance are unavailable, are contraindicated or is not possible, as in newborns.

Course of Recovery

Barbiturate overdose recovery is somewhat similar to recovery from alcohol overdose. There occurs an initial rapid improvement and reduction in intoxication following treatment. This may be followed by nausea, weakness, anxiety, tremors, abdominal cramps and vomiting. In chronic heavy users, the symptoms may begin from 1½ to 5 days after the last dose, manifested as seizures. Delirium tremens may develop 3–7 days after the last dose.

Benzodiazepines are the mainstay of treatment for these symptoms. However, sometimes the patients are refractory to treatment with these drugs.

Complications

1. Acute pneumonia.
2. Renal failure.
3. Pulmonary edema.
4. Hypotension.
5. Respiratory depression.

SALICYLATES

SALICYLATE POISONING IN CHILDREN

Aspirin poisoning is common in children, especially in toddlers in whom accidental poisoning can easily occur. Salicylates are present in many OTC drugs to be used as anti-inflammatory in soft tissue, joint diseases and vasculitis like acute rheumatic fever, Kawasaki disease, etc. or pain killers for muscle and joint pain. It has mild antipyretic properties and can be used as an antithrombotic medication. Salicylates are available in several forms, as liquids, tablets, caplets and as topical application creams and gels. The gels usually consist of methyl salicylate, which has a pungent odor, yet is accidentally consumed by children. It is usually a concentrated form, each teaspoon of methyl salicylate consisting of nearly 7,000 mg of salicylate, which is at least 4 times the lethal dose of salicylate in children. Some herbal preparations also contain salicylate, hence parents must be aware of its potential toxicity, while utilizing these products.

The incidence of salicylate poisoning has reduced in children, due to the drug being replaced by paracetamol/acetaminophen as an antipyretic-analgesic. However, accidental ingestion in children continues to occur, while in adolescents the suicidal behavior increases the likelihood of toxicity.

What happens when excess Aspirin is ingested?

Once the Aspirin is ingested and reaches the stomach, it disintegrates and dissolves. The acetyl group from the acetylsalicylic acid is split and is inactivated by the plasma esterases, while the salicylate gets absorbed and widely distributed in the body, entering the intra and extracellular spaces. At therapeutic doses, the salicylic acid is metabolized in the liver and excreted in 2–3 hours.

In toxic doses, the salicylates have complex effects on the various organ systems. They uncouple the oxidative phosphorylation, inhibit the Krebs cycle enzymes and inhibit the amino acid synthesis. The citric acid cycle is also inhibited, which along with the uncoupling of the oxidative phosphorylation can result in renal insufficiency, with accumulation of sulfuric acid and phosphoric acid. Fatty acid metabolism is abnormal, with resultant ketone body formation. All these processes result in an increased anion-gap metabolic acidosis. The respiratory center is directly stimulated by the salicylate, resulting in primary respiratory alkalosis. This combination of primary respiratory alkalosis, with primary metabolic acidosis, is the classical feature of acute salicylate toxicity (Fig. 4.3).

Toxic Dose of Salicylate

The amount of salicylate ingested may help to assess the potential toxicity and morbidity in cases of overdose. This, however acts as a rough guide in cases of acute salicylate poisoning:

1. Below 150 mg/kg: no toxicity to mild toxicity.
2. From 150 to 300 mg/kg: mild-to-moderate toxicity.
3. From 301 to 500 mg/kg: severe toxicity.
4. Greater than 500 mg/kg: potentially lethal dose.

Symptoms

An accurate history is very important to aid the diagnosis. In the history, it is essential to determine the amount of salicylate ingested, the type or the preparation of the drug, the timing of ingestion any potential coingestants and any underlying disease conditions. All these need to be documented, as they can act as a guide to the treatment regimen. Tinnitus is a valuable symptom of salicylate poisoning. Tachycardia, tachypnea, hyperpyrexia are commonly associated symptoms.

Signs

Salicylates affect various organ systems in the body and accordingly produce varying physical signs. The physician has to be alert to notice and recognize the various signs, so as to provide appropriate and timely treatment (Fig. 4.4).

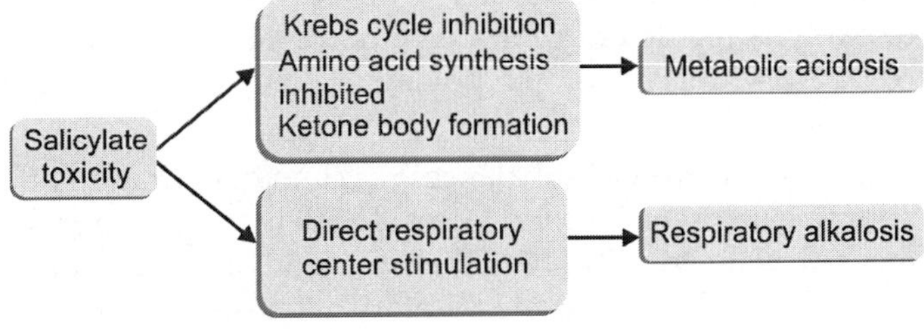

Fig. 4.3: Metabolic derangements in salicylate toxicity

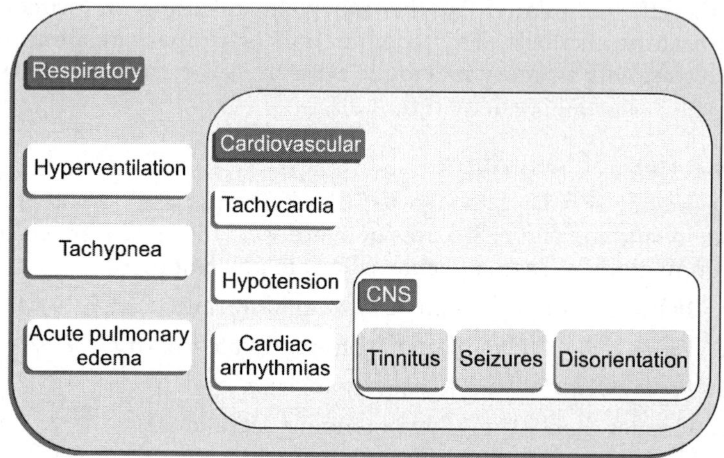

Fig. 4.4: Common signs of salicylate poisoning

1. Respiratory system—the salicylates cause both direct and indirect stimulation of the respiratory center, resulting in tachypnea and hyperpnea. It can also give rise to non-cardiogenic pulmonary edema and acute lung injury. All this can manifest as hyperventilation, hyperpnea and respiratory distress with resultant respiratory arrest. Fever can also give rise to hyperpnea and may be associated with aspiration pneumonitis.
2. Cardiovascular—tachycardia with minimal cardiac compromise may occur. However, it may also cause hypotension, possibly secondary to the cardiac arrthymias that may occur. Ventricular tachycardia, ventricular fibrillations, premature ventricular contractions, etc. which can ultimately result in asystole, especially with severe toxicity. Sudden hemodynamic deterioration commonly occurs secondary to respiratory depression. Hypokalemia may occur due to the toxicity.
3. Fluid and electrolyte imbalances result in dehydration due to vomiting or insensible fluid losses. The dehydration aggravates the salicylate toxicity. Hypokalemia and hypocalcemia can occur due to the primary respiratory alkalosis.

4. Gastrointestinal effects—nausea and vomiting, which may be due to the direct effect of the salicylate on the gastric mucosa, pylorospasm can occur, which can slow down the GI motility and hence increase the salicylate absorption from the GIT. Severe toxicity can result in GI bleeds.
5. Salicylates produce thromboxane A2, which can together with the inhibited Vit. K-dependent enzymes, result in bleeding. Salicylates also cause hypoprothrombinemia and dysfunctional platelets, which can also aggravate the bleeding tendencies.
6. Hepatic disease in the form of acute hepatitis or Reye's syndrome can be precipitated by the salicylate toxicity. Liver enzymes are elevated and there may be fatty infiltration of the liver, leading to fulminant hepatitis, coma and death.
7. Musculoskeletal damage in the form of rhabdomyolysis due to the uncoupling of the oxidative phosphorylation and the resultant dissipation of heat and energy.
8. Central nervous system effects—salicylates are directly neurotoxic and is directly related to the amount of drug ingested. As the blood pH drops towards acidity, the non-ionized drug easily crosses the blood-brain barrier and exerts effects on the CNS. Tinnitus is one of the early symptoms of CNS effects. Severe hearing loss, blurring of vision and deafness can occur with higher doses of toxicity. The other CNS effects, include nausea, vomiting, lethargy, hyperventilation. Continued, severe toxicity could result in disorientation, cardiorespiratory depression, hyperthermia, seizures and eventually death. CNS encephalopathy associated with hallucinations, confusion, irritability and hyperactivity can occur in severe toxicity.
9. Genitourinary—acute renal failure may occur as a primary response to salicylate toxicity or could occur secondary to multiorgan failure.
10. Dermatologic features are generally secondary to contact dermatitis with salicylate containing preparations.

Laboratory Investigations

1. Blood levels of salicylate—levels between 15 and 30 mg/dL are therapeutic. Levels begin to rise after 4–6 hours following

ingestion. Signs and symptoms appear at levels 30 mg/dL. Levels of 100 mg/dL are potentially lethal and need urgent hemodialysis. Levels need to be measured every 2 hours until peaking occurs, then every 4–6 hourly until the levels decrease to the non-toxic range.

2. Serum electrolytes—potassium, calcium, magnesium and glucose levels need to be monitored at least every 12th hourly. In case of alkalinization of the urine, the serum potassium levels need to be very closely monitored.
3. Serum creatinine and blood urea nitrogen (BUN)—levels need to be monitored to watch for signs of acute renal failure. Levels need to be repeated every 12 hours.
4. Urine exam—urine pH to be checked and closely monitored, especially during alkalinization therapy. Maintain urine pH between 7.5 and 8. Urine can also be tested for a toxicology screen.
5. Urine ferric chloride test—is a bedside test to detect the presence of salicylate in the urine. Add a few drops of 10% ferric chloride to a 1 mL sample of urine and look for color change. A persistent purple color will indicate the presence of salicylate in the urine. This test gives an immediate result, but is not useful to estimate the salicylate levels, hence is replaced by the serum level estimations.
6. Arterial blood gas (ABG) analysis—is essential to be monitored as the acid-base disturbances are likely to develop after salicylate toxicity.
7. Chest X-ray—to be taken in case of suspected pulmonary edema, aspiration pneumonia or hypoxemia.
8. Abdominal X-ray to be taken in case of suspected salicylate concretions or bezoars. This is to be suspected, when the salicylate levels do not decrease despite adequate treatment or the patient's condition continues to deteriorate despite treatment.
9. Miscellaneous investigations:
   a. CBC—altered levels could give an indication of superadded infection, aspiration pneumonitis, etc.
   b. Prothrombin time and activated partial thromboplastin time (APTT)—will be indicative of hemorrhagic tendency.

c. Liver function tests—indicates the status of the liver functions affected due to toxicity.
d. Abdominal USG/CT—in case of suspected bezoars, which cannot be detected by the X-rays.

Treatment

No specific antidote for salicylate poisoning. Administer supportive treatment to the patient immediately as follows:

1. Airway maintenance: Assess the adequacy of the airway and respiration, administer supplemental oxygen. If altered sensorium, intubate the patient and provide assisted ventilation. Continuous monitoring of the airway status is essential to check for any deterioration in the patient's condition.
2. Check the body temperature, if possible the rectal temperature to gauge the core temperature. If hypothermic, carefully rewarm the patient.
3. Administer IV fluids and aggressively treat the hypovolemic shock. If the shock persists despite aggressive fluid replacement, administer vasopressors, e.g. dopamine, IV (dose: 5–10 µg/kg/min as continuous infusion).
4. Irrigate the exposed part like skin or eyes with water to thoroughly wash away any traces of salicylate that could be present.
5. Gastric decontamination: To be done after the patient is stabilized.
   a. Gastric lavage to be done, after ensuring the protection of the airway.
   b. Can be performed, if the patient is seen within 60 minutes of ingestion of the drug.
   c. Activated charcoal helps to limit the further absorption of the salicylate via the gastric mucosa. Initial dose is 1 g/kg body weight of activated charcoal, up to a maximum of 50 mg. Repeated doses of activated charcoal may be useful to help in elimination of the salicylates from the circulation into the GIT and hence assist in the elimination.
   d. Whole bowel irrigation using polyethylene glycol is more useful than single dose administration of activated charcoal for the elimination of salicylate from the circulation.

6. Urine elimination.
   a. Administer fluids for fluid deficit correction, which will enhance elimination of the salicylate from the circulation. Administer Ringer's lactate 10–20 mL/kg/h till the urine output of 1–1.5 mL/kg/h is achieved.
   b. Alkalinization of the urine helps in the elimination of the salicylate. When the urine pH is raised to 8, the clearance of the salicylate increases at least 10–20 fold, thereby decreasing the half-life of the salicylate to around 8 hours. The salicylate is a weak acid, which ionizes on exposure to the alkali and these ions are poorly reabsorbed by the tubules, hence they are readily excreted in the urine. An initial bolus of 1 mEq/kg of sodium bicarbonate is administered, followed by a continuous infusion, which runs at twice the maintenance requirements, along with titration of the urine pH to above 7.5.

To prepare the fluid: Use 0.5 normal saline or 5% dextrose to which add 50–150 mEq of sodium bicarbonate per liter of the fluid, resulting in an isotonic fluid.

Rate of administration of the fluid: 1–2 L/h.

Once the urine output has been established, administer 20–40 mEq/L of KCl , to prevent the occurrence of hypokalemia, which can inhibit the elimination of the salicylate in the urine. Potassium needs to be administered, even when the serum potassium level is in the low normal range, to promote adequate ionization of the salicylate. Continue the alkalinization until the serum salicylate reaches the therapeutic levels of 30 mg/dL.

7. Hemodialysis—is preferred to the other methods of dialysis, as the elimination of the drug is more efficient and effective.

   Indications for hemodialysis:
   a. Refractory acidosis.
   b. Severe electrolyte imbalance.
   c. Serum levels above 100–120 mg/dL.
   d. Non-cardiogenic pulmonary edema.
   e. Volume overload.
   f. Seizures.

g. Coma.
h. Renal failure.

Indications for Discharge

1. Serum salicylate levels at therapeutic levels—30 mg/dL.
2. No acid-base disturbance.
3. Gastric decontamination completed.
4. Patient is stable.

Prognosis

Prognosis is good when the patient is stable, no signs of toxicity are noted and the serum levels are in the normal range. The patient must be protected against repeated exposure to accidental toxicity from any drug. In case of intentional drug overdose, the patient needs to be seen by a psychiatrist for counseling and guidance.

TRICYCLIC ANTIDEPRESSANTS

TRICYCLIC ANTIDEPRESSANTS POISONING IN CHILDREN

Tricyclic antidepressants are currently termed as cyclic antideppressants, as some newer members of this group have a 4-ring structure. This class of drugs is used in children to treat forms of school phobia, obsessive-compulsive disorders, attention deficit hyperactivity disorders, separation anxiety, as well as the treatment of enuresis. The common drugs in this group include amitriptyline, imipramine, desipramine, nortriptyline, doxepin and clomipramine.

Pathophysiology

Cyclic antidepressants have a narrow therapeutic window. They are rapidly absorbed in the GIT and undergo first pass metabolism in the liver, where they are conjugated and then excreted via the kidneys. They are lipophilic and extensively protein bound, leading to large volumes of distribution. The elimination half-life is over 24 hours and in cases of overdose, the elimination may be prolonged and can aggravate the toxic effects.

The cyclic antidepressants have anticholinergic effects. They also decrease the central norepinephrine and serotonin reuptake with resultant increase in the levels of biogenic amines in the brain. In addition, it also has direct alpha-adrenergic effects and has a stabilizing effect on the myocardial membrane cells by blocking the fast sodium channels located there.

CNS effects and cardiovascular instability are the predominant adverse effects and as the level of the biogenic amine rises, the likelihood of seizures also increases. Impaired cardiovascular conduction with widened QRS complexes, prolonged QT and PR intervals and decreased slope of phase zero depolarization can result in heart block and unstable ventricular arrhythmias, which may also lead to asystole. Vasodilatation due to alpha-adrenergic blockade causes profound hypotension, which can be life-threatening.

Symptoms and Signs

The effects of signs and symptoms are as follows:

1. CVS effects
   a. Hypotension.

b. Sinus tachycardia.
c. Peripheral vasodilatation.
d. Ventricular arrhythmias.
e. Prolonged PR, QRS, QT.
f. Intervals.
g. Cardiogenic shock.
h. Asystole.

2. CNS effects
   a. Drowsiness.
   b. Rigidity.
   c. Extrapyramidal signs.
   d. Ophthalmoplegia.
   e. Respiratory depression.
   f. Delirium.
   g. Seizures.
   h. Coma.
3. Anticholinergic effects
   a. Pyrexia.
   b. Blurred vision, mydriasis.
   c. Muscle twitching.
   d. Xerostomia.
   e. Absent bowel sounds.
   f. Urinary retention.

Important Signs

- **S**—Shock
- **A**—Altered mental status
- **L**—Long QRS interval
- **T**—Terminal R wave in aVR.

Investigations

1. Routine CBC and urinalysis.
2. Serum potassium levels: Hypokalemia due to norepinephrine blockade and resultant catecholamine stimulation, which in turn has adverse cardiac effects.

3. Renal function tests: Abnormal renal functions can aggravate the toxic effects of the pharmacologically active metabolites that are produced by the hepatic metabolism of cyclic antidepressants.
4. Arterial blood gases: Respiratory depression together with myocardial depression and peripheral vasodilatation can cause hypotension and increased lactate production. Thus, there is a mixed acidosis, which decreases the protein binding of the drug, with increased in the free drug levels and aggravated toxicity.
5. Toxicology screen: Serum levels of cyclic antidepressants will aid the diagnosis. However, the levels are not an accurate indicator, due to the extensive protein binding of the drug, with diffuse tissue distribution.
6. Chest X-ray: To rule out the other causes of respiratory depression and to rule out aspiration.
7. ECG in all leads: Can be used as a screening tool for cyclic depressant toxicity, as well as a prognostic indicator. Widened QRS complexes can be used to prognosticate the occurrence of seizures and arrhythmias. The right fascicle is predominantly affected, with an elevated R wave in the lead aVR. The amplitude of the R wave could be predictive of seizures and arrhythmias.

Treatment

1. Initial stabilization of the patient—check ABC and stabilize. Algorithm for treatment is shown in Figure 4.5.
2. If patient presents early, within 1 hour of toxin consumption, there is a role for gastric lavage. Always anticipate the deterioration in condition of the symptomatic patients. Hence, it is recommended to intubate the patient before performing the gastric lavage.
3. Elective intubation is indicated in patients with poor cardiopulmonary reserve, those with impending respiratory failure and patients who are obtunded and mentally not alert.
4. Intravenous fluids as bolus to treat the hypotension. In case of refractory hypotension, administer pressor agents, preferably those with alpha-adrenergic action. Dopamine should not be used, as its action depends on release of norepinephrine levels, which may be decreased due to the blockade by

the overdosed cyclic antidepressants. Epinephrine is indicated in these cases, as it gives better response with lesser chances of arrhythmias.

5. Cardiac monitoring to be started early and continued for at least 6–8 hours. Usually the dysrhythmias present early, within 1–2 hours of ingestion. In patients with evidence of dysrhythmias, the cardiac monitoring should be continued for at least 24 hours after the normalization of the ECG patterns.
6. In case of urinary retention due to the anticholinergic actions, insert a Foley catheter and relieve the bladder obstruction.
7. In case of seizures, administer benzodiazepines. Diazepam or Lorazepam are effective by depressing all levels of the CNS, induced by increased levels of GABA, which is the major inhibitory neurotransmitter at all levels of the CNS.
8. In case of acidosis, administer sodium bicarbonate to maintain the pH between 7.45 and 7.55. This helps to decrease the

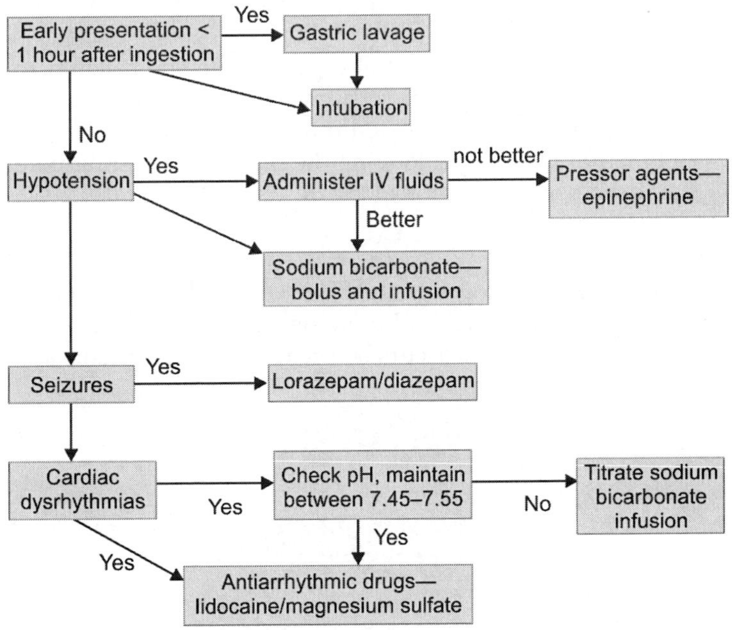

Fig. 4.5: Algorithm for treatment of tricyclic antidepressant poisoning

occurrence of cardiac dysrhythmias, stabilze the arrhythmias if any, decrease the QRS interval and increase the blood pressure. Start infusion with 1–2 mEq/kg bolus and follow with a maintenance infusion that maintains the pH below 7.55 and the QRS width of 100 milliseconds. The QTc interval also needs to be monitored, as the sodium bicarbonate can cause prolongation of the QTc interval.

9. Treatment of cardiac arrhythmias: Most of the dysrhythmias caused by tricyclic antidepressant overdose is corrected by the administration of sodium bicarbonate and alkalinization of the serum. In resistant cases with persistent dysrhythmias, use of lidocaine and magnesium sulfate has been found to correct the cardiac rhythm. Always alkalinize the serum before use of the antiarrhythmic drugs.

   Lidocaine acts by elevating the stimulation threshold of the ventricles and suppressing the conduction through the tissues. Administer loading dose 1 mg/kg, which can be repeated every 5 minutes for 3 doses maximum and follow-up with a maintenance infusion of 15–50 μg/kg/min.

   Magnesium sulfate acts by preventing the calcium flux and also activates the sodium-potassium ATPase, thus affecting the transport of sodium and potassium across the cell membrane and prolonging the membrane resting potential. Used as 50% solution at the dose of 0.05–0.1 mL/kg IV.

Prognosis

Early arrival and appropriate treatment in hospital is associated with good prognosis, the fatality being around 1%–2%. Most of the mortality, almost 70% occurs before the patient presents at the hospital for treatment.

THEOPHYLLINE

THEOPHYLLINE POISONING IN CHILDREN

Theophylline belongs to the group of methylxanthines. It can directly stimulate the beta-1 as well as the beta-2 receptors via the release of endogenous catecholamines.

Theophylline is used as a bronchodilator in the treatment of asthma in children. It is also used in neonates for the treatment of apnea. In adults, it is used in the treatment of chronic obstructive pulmonary disease (COPD). In recent times, its use in the treatment of childhood asthma has considerably decreased. However, it is still available as a component with other bronchodilators in several preparations. Theophylline has a narrow safety window and this can be further decreased by the effects of other medications, diet and underlying disease, giving rise to the possibility of toxic symptoms even with therapeutic doses of the drug.

Pathophysiology

Theophylline acts by blocking adenosine production, which decreases the levels of histamine in the body and hence can reverse the brochospasm. Theophylline also acts as a phosphodiesterase inhibitor, resulting in elevated levels of cyclic adenosine monophosphate and adrenergic stimulation.

Theophylline is rapidly and completely absorbed on oral administration and peak levels are reached within 30–120 minutes. It has a half-life of 4–6 hours, which may be higher in case of overdose. On IV administration, peak levels are achieved within 30 minutes. Theophylline is excreted by the cytochrome P450 system and a small quantity is excreted in the urine. Drugs like cimetidine, erythromycin and oral contraceptives, which interfere with the cytochrome P450 enzymes can prolong the duration of action of the drug in the body.

1. Therapeutic dose: 10–20 μg/mL.
2. Toxic dose: greater than 20 μg/mL.
3. Lethal dose: 80–100 μg/mL.

Symptoms

With acute toxicity, the GIT symptoms predominate.

- Nausea
- Vomiting can be protracted
- Intractable thirst
- Abdominal pain
- Diarrhea
- Tremors, restlessness
- Hallucinations
- Headache
- Irritability
- Convulsions
- Cardiac arrhythmias.

Signs

Classified according to the different systems involved.

1. GIT:
    a. Vomiting.
    b. Abdominal pain.
    c. Diarrhea.
2. Cardiac:
    a. Cardiac arrhythmias.
        i. Sinus tachycardia.
        ii. Supraventricular tachycardia.
        iii. Multifocal atrial tachycardia.
        iv. Atrial fibrillation.
        v. Atrial flutter.
        vi. Ventricular tachycardia.
        vii. Ventricular fibrillation.
    b. Pulseless electrical activity.
    c. Hypotension.
    d. Cardiac arrest.

3. CNS:
   a. Restlessness.
   b. Tremors.
   c. Agitation.
   d. Seizures.
   e. Hallucinations.
4. Pulmonary:
   a. Increased respiratory rate.
   b. Respiratory alkalosis.
   c. Acute lung injury.
   d. Respiratory failure.
   e. Respiratory arrest.

Investigations

1. CBC—can show elevated WBC count due to increased catecholamine activity.
2. Blood glucose levels—may show hyperglycemia.
3. Serum electrolytes—evaluate for the following:
   a. Hypokalemia.
   b. Hypercalcemia.
   c. Hypocalcemia.
   d. Hypophosphatemia.
   e. Ketosis.
   f. Metabolic acidosis.
4. Serum theophylline levels: to be closely monitored. Some preparations are sustained release, hence elevated levels may continue for several hours. Repeat levels every 2 hours till normalcy.
5. Serum levels of acetaminophen and aspirin to be checked.
6. ECG in all 12 leads—to act as a baseline measure of cardiac function as well as to look for any associated cardiac dysrhythmias, electrolyte abnormality, etc.
7. Lumbar puncture—to evaluate recent onset seizures.
8. CT scan brain—in case of recurrent seizures, altered mental status and to rule out any associated CNS pathology.

Treatment

1. Assess the airway status. If patient is in altered sensory or respiratory distress, intubate and secure the airway.
2. Administer oxygen after measuring the SpO_2 levels.
3. Insert venous cannula to maintain the IV line and in case the necessity for hemoperfusion arises. Administer IV fluids. In case of hypotension, use Ringer's lactate at 10–20 mL/kg/h. If no hypotension, administer maintenance fluids.
4. Abort the seizures, in case the patient is having convulsions.
5. In case of persistent vomiting, administer IV ondansetron.
6. Gastric lavage is indicated if:
   a. The patient has presented within 1 hour of consumption.
   b. In case of consumption of sustained release form of theophylline.
   c. In case of suspicion of theophylline bezoar formation.

   Activated charcoal is administered to adsorb the ingested theophylline. Repeated doses may need to be administered in order to facilitate the drug expulsion. Ensure that the patient is able to protect his airway to reduce the risk of aspiration.

   Sorbitol may be administered once along with the activated charcoal to ensure complete bowel emptying.
7. In case of poisoning with sustained release preparations, whole bowel irrigation may be required, to ensure complete elimination. Administer polyethylene glycol at 500 mL/h, until the rectal effluent is clear.
8. Correction of underlying electrolyte abnormalities:
   a. Hypokalemia.
   b. Hypocalcemia.
   c. Hypophosphatemia.
9. Treatment of seizures: The patient may present with convulsions and medication needs to be administered immediately to abort the seizure. Benzodiazepines, either diazepam or lorazepam, is to be administered immediately. These drugs can also help to decrease the associated anxiety and restlessness.

Phenobarbitones are used as prophylaxis to prevent the occurrence of seizures, in those at high risk of having seizures. This includes:

a. Patients with high levels of theophylline greater than 80 μg/mL.
b. Patients younger than 3 years of age.
c. Patients with chronic toxicity having levels greater than 40 μg/mL.

Phenobarbitones have the added advantage of increasing the hepatic metabolism of theophylline and hence increased drug excretion. However, they can also precipitate hypotension, hence care must be taken to maintain adequate fluid infusion.

10. In case of hypotension, despite adequate IV fluids, administer vasopressors, especially with alpha-adrenergic receptor activity like phenylephrine or norepinephrine. Use beta blockers with care, especially with underlying bronchospastic disease. If beta blockers are needed, esmolol is preferred to the others, as it is short acting.
11. In case of unstable supraventricular tachycardia (SVT), administer beta blockers, preferably esmolol, with caution for its negative inotropic effects which may precipitate hypotension.
12. Hemoperfusion with charcoal is indicated when:
    a. Symptomatic patient, with levels greater than 90 μg/mL.
    b. Hypotension not responding to IV fluid correction.
    c. Recurrent or persistent seizures.
    d. Chronic toxicity with theophylline level greater than 40 μg/mL.
    e. Ventricular dysrhythmia.
13. Hemodialysis may be performed in case facilities for hemoperfusion are unavailable and the patient's condition warrants immediate corrective measures.

Prognosis

Complete recovery occurs in case of early and adequate treat-ment. The patient and family needs to be counseled before discharge. Drug safety methods need to be explained to the family members.

SUGGESTED READING

Paracetamol Toxicity in Children

1. Farrell SE. Acetaminophen toxicity. www.medscape.com [Accessed May, 2012].
2. Goldstein RJ. Hydrocarbons toxicity treatment and management. www.medscape.com [Accessed May, 2012].
3. Kleigman RM, Behrman RE, Jenson HB, et al. Nelson Textbook of Pediatrics, 18th edition. Elsevier Health Sciences Division; 2007.
4. Penna A, Buchanar N. Paracetamol poisoning in children and hepatotoxicity. Br J Clinical Pharmacol. 1991;32(2):143-49.

Non-steroidal Anti-inflammatory Drugs

1. Kleigman RM, Behrman RE, Jenson HB, et al. Nelson Textbook of Pediatrics, 18th edition. Elsevier Health Sciences Division; 2007.
2. Vale JA, Meredith TJ. Acute poisoning due to non-steroidal anti-inflammatory drugs. Med Toxicol. 1986;1(1):12-31.
3. Wiegand TJ, Tarabar A. Non-steroidal anti-inflammatory agent toxicity. www.medscape.com [Accessed May, 2012].

Barbiturates

1. Burns MJ, Schwartzstein. Enhanced elimination of poisons. www.medscape.com [Accessed May, 2012].
2. Kleigman RM, Behrman RE, Jenson HB, et al. Nelson Textbook of Pediatrics, 18th edition. Elsevier Health Sciences Division; 2007.
3. Proudfoot AT, Krenzelok EP, Vale JA. Position paper on urine alkalinization. Clin Toxicol. 2004;42(1):1-26.
4. Shashikiran. Management of barbiturate poisoning—a case report. Indian J Anaesth. 2002;46(6):480-82.

Salicylates

1. Kleigman RM, Behrman RE, Jenson HB, et al. Nelson Textbook of Pediatrics, 18th edition. Elsevier Health Sciences Division; 2007.
2. Poirier R, Corbet R, Salicylate poisoning in children. Can Med Assoc J. 1952;67(2):117-20.

Tricyclic Antidepressants

1. Kleigman RM, Behrman RE, Jenson HB, et al. Nelson Textbook of Pediatrics, 18th edition. Elsevier Health Sciences Division; 2007.
2. Rashida Y White-McCrimmon. Tricyclic Antidepressant Toxicity in Pediatrics. www.medscape.com

Theophylline

1. Greg Hymel MD. In: Asim Tarabar MD (Ed). Theophylline Toxicity in Emergency Medicine. www.medscape.com
2. Kleigman RM, Behrman RE, Jenson HB, et al. Nelson Textbook of Pediatrics, 18th edition. Elsevier Health Sciences Division; 2007.

5 Chapter Metals

IRON

IRON POISONING

Iron poisoning is a common condition in children, as the iron tablets are easily mistaken for candy and peppermints by the children.

Fatal Dose of Iron in Children

1. For children below 5 years of age, 250 mg of elemental iron is the fatal dose.
2. Dose:
   a. 20 mg/kg elemental iron can cause mild symptoms of toxicity.
   b. 40 mg/kg elemental iron can result in moderate intoxication.
   c. 60 mg/kg elemental iron can be fatal.
3. In older children, 900 mg of elemental iron can be fatal.

Pathophysiology

Local effects: Local corrosive action of the iron on the gastrointestinal (GI) mucosal membrane causes the breakdown of the mucosal barrier, which could result in vomiting, massive GI hemorrhage and bleeding. The patient can become hypovolemic due to the large fluid losses. Large amounts of iron can get absorbed and result in metabolic damage.

Cellular toxicity: Once absorbed, the iron gets deposited in various organs of the body and exerts metabolic effects. There occurs altered oxidative phosphorylation and mitochondrial dysfunction resulting in cellular death. The liver is the most affected, but other organs like heart, kidneys and hematologic systems may also be affected.

Both the corrosive actions and the cellular toxicity of iron overload could result in metabolic dysfunction, particularly metabolic acidosis.

Lactic acidosis results from vasodilatation and the negative ionotropic effect of iron and the volume loss, which induces hypoperfusion.

As the oxidative phosphorylation is inhibited, there occurs anaerobic metabolism, which again aggravates the metabolic acidosis.

Signs and Symptoms of Iron Toxicity

Following excessive iron ingestion, the child may pass through four stages. At each stage, the signs and symptoms are different and any stage may be fatal, if appropriate care is not taken, else it may progress to the next stage of severity.

Stage 1: Early Stage (GI Stage)

First stage may be noted soon after the excessive iron ingestion. It is the stage of local GI irritation at the site of contact of the iron tablets. It is characterized by local necrosis and GI hemorrhage.

At this stage, the child complains of abdominal pain, nausea, vomiting and diarrhea. Hematemesis and melena may occur depending on the severity of GI irritation.

This stage starts immediately and could last up to 6 hours postingestion.

In very severe cases, fluid and blood loss may occur into the GI lumen and the child may end up with shock. Lethargy, convulsions and coma may also occur at this stage. Shock and coma in stage 1 carry a very poor prognosis.

Stage 2: Latent Stage

Second stage is the stage of apparent recovery and improvement. This stage lasts for 6–12 hours postingestion. The apparent recovery may be due to the distribution of the ingested iron to the various body tissues.

At this stage, iron absorption continues from the GI tract (GIT), but it starts depositing in various organs of the body, especially the liver, wherein it starts accumulating inside and damaging the mitochondria of the cells.

In cases of mild toxicity, complete recovery may occur at this stage. In other cases, the patient may progress to stage 3 directly. Signs at this stage may be very mild—tachycardia, lethargy or tachypnea may occur.

Stage 3: Metabolic/Cardiovascular Stage

Third stage begins after 12–24 hours following ingestion of the iron overdose. Most deaths occur at this stage. It is the stage of multisystem damage.

This is the stage of metabolic abnormalities. Prothrombin time (PT) is prolonged, aspartate aminotransferase (AST), alanine aminotransferase (ALT) are deranged and hypoglycemia may occur. Coagulopathy, shock seizures and altered mental status may be noted. Metabolic acidosis may occur at this stage.

Stage 4: Hepatic Stage

Fourth stage occurs 2–3 days after ingestion. This stage is characterized by extensive liver damage. The liver function tests are abnormal.

Stage 5: Late Stage/Delayed Stage

Fifth stage occurs 2–6 weeks postexposure. At this stage, the late GI effects of the iron injury is observed in the form of scarring and pyloric stenosis, pyloric obstruction, hepatic cirrhosis. This stage is rare, even in cases of severe poisoning. However, in cases of severe obstruction, surgical relief of the obstruction may be essential.

The sequelae of GI irritation that has occurred in stage 1 is seen in the form of scarring and pyloric stenosis. The extent of the sequelae depends on the extent of initial GI damage. The pyloric stenosis may require surgical correction.

Investigations

1. History of ingestion of iron tablets.
2. Plain abdominal X-ray: may show the radiopaque iron tablets, if taken before the disintegration of the tablets.
3. Gastric lavage fluid or collected vomitus may reveal the ingested iron tablets. If tablets are not visible as such, the lavage fluid or the vomitus can be subjected to a simple chemical analysis, which may show evidence of iron.

a. Dilute and filter the lavage fluid/vomitus.
b. Take 5 mL of filtrate and add 1 mL of 10% potassium ferricyanide. An intense color reaction with Prussian blue color is noted with even traces of ferrous sulfate.
c. Take 5 mL of the filtrate and add 1 mL of 10% potassium ferrocyanide. A color change of the filtrate to produce blue color indicates the presence of the ferric form of iron, which could have been formed due to the gastric conversion of the iron compound.

4. Serum iron levels: Levels over 5 mg/mL indicate elevated blood levels. However, severe iron poisoning could occur in the absence of elevated serum levels, as the iron may be deposited in the liver immediately after absorption. Serum levels of iron are not an accurate guide to the extent of poisoning, as the levels could vary depending on the time of collection after ingestion. Elevated levels may occur early, soon after ingestion.
5. Therapeutic trial: Single dose of deferoxamine 1 g intramuscular (IM) or intravenous (IV) is given and the color of the urine is noted. Colorless urine could indicate minimum/no toxicity.

   Pink or red color urine: Indicates severe iron toxicity. The ingested excess iron, after saturation of the serum transferring, is present as free iron in the serum. This combines with the Desferal to produce an iron-chelate feroxamine, which has a pink color and appears in the urine.

Treatment

Emergency Treatment

To be given to unstable patients with signs of acute toxicity:

1. Intravenous (IV) access to be established.
2. In case of hypovolemia, administer IV fluids rapidly 20 mL/kg over 30 minutes of Ringer's lactate or 0.9% sodium chloride.
3. Oxygen inhalation in case of shock.

Therapy for Iron Toxicity

Once a diagnosis of iron toxicity has been established, it is essential to start early definitive treatment, to avoid the deposition of the iron in the liver and other tissues. Once iron deposition has oc-curred in the hepatic mitochondria, it is an irreversible condition.

The aim of treatment is two fold:

1. To prevent and reduce the further absorption of iron from the GIT.
2. To prevent iron accumulation in the liver.

Prevention of further absorption of iron from the GIT: Decontamination—induce emesis before gastric lavage. This will remove the large fragments of the iron tablets, which may block the lavage tube. Plain abdominal X-ray may be taken before emesis, which may reveal the radiopaque iron tablets.

Gastric lavage as soon as possible using 1% sodium bicarbonate, containing 2 g/L of deferoxamine (4 vials of Desferal/L). Sodium bicarbonate is used to maintain the gastric pH around 5 at which level, the iron converts to the ferric form and is easier to chelate with deferoxamine.

Chelation of iron

Iron chelation is the mainstay of treatment, as it prevents further iron absorption and deposition in the various body organs. Symptoms of iron toxicity and serum levels of iron are only rough guides for the requirements of chelation. However, levels of 350 μg/mL in patients with symptoms and 500 μg/mL without symptoms would indicate requirement for chelation therapy.

Deferoxamine (Desferal) is the drug of choice for chelation in case of iron toxicity. It chelates the free iron and the iron bound to ferritin and hemosiderin, to form feroxamine, which is not absorbed and is excreted in the urine, giving a pink coloration to the urine. It is given as a continuous IV infusion to give the best result, but may also be given IM or slow IV, especially in cases of severe toxicity with hypovolemia and collapse, where the IV route is preferred.

Presentation of Desferal: Available as lyophilized substance in vials containing 500 mg per vial. To be diluted with 2 mL of sterile water to form 250 mg/mL, which can be used for IM injections. For IV injection, it may be dissolved in normal saline, Ringer's lactate or dextrose saline.

Dose: Four vials (2 g) are given stat IM along with gastric lavage. This could be followed by continuous IV infusion at a rate of 15 mg/kg/h (maximum dose of 80 mg/kg/24 h).

Repeat dose of 2 g of Desferal may be given IM after 12 hours.

Duration of treatment: No clear-cut-end-point, but as long as the urine color remains pink, it indicates continued iron chelation and excretion. Serum levels of iron may guide the duration of treatment.

LEAD

LEAD POISONING IN CHILDREN

Lead is an element that is found in many sources in nature. However, toxicity results from the long-standing exposure to particular lead containing compounds.

Lead poisoning is invariably a chronic toxicity, as it takes several years for the symptom complex to develop and manifest in the child.

Sources of Lead

There are two important sources of lead (Fig. 5.1):

1. Airborne lead—from the combustion of tetraethyl lead in gasoline.
2. Ingested lead—dust and chips from bits of lead paint.

Lead from the gasoline can settle in the soil, which can also get contaminated by chips and bits of lead paint, from peeling walls and plaster.

Other sources of lead are:

1. Water that comes in lead pipes is usually a source of lead contamination.
2. Toys usually are colored with paints that contain lead.

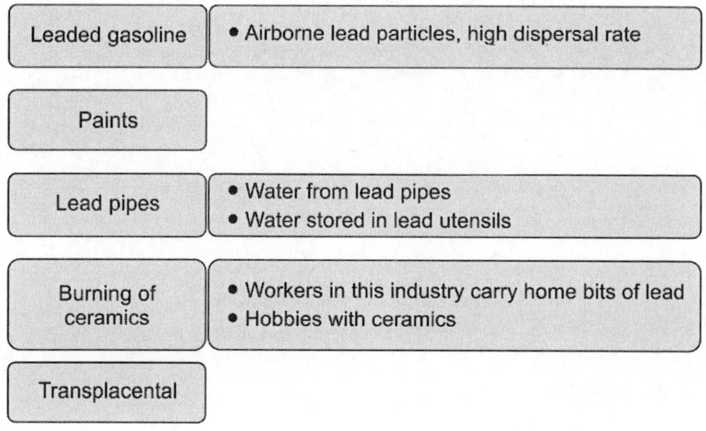

Fig. 5.1: Sources of lead

3. Burning of ceramics, paints and other lead containing articles.
4. Transplacental transfer.
5. Transfer of lead via breast milk in infants.

Pathophysiology

Lead interferes with various enzymatic functions and impairs their actions. Lead alters very basic nervous system functions, such as calcium-modulated signaling. Lead interferes detectably with heme synthesis beginning at blood lead concentrations of approximately 25 μg/dL. Both aminolevulinate dehydratase, an early step enzyme and ferrochelatase, which completes the heme ring, are inhibited by lead.

Signs and Symptoms

Usually, the early symptoms are subtle and need to be carefully watched.

1. Anemia—subtle signs, impaired cognition, pallor disproportionate to the degree of anemia.
2. Lead colic—abdominal pain, which is not localized, constipation, occasional vomiting.
3. Lead line on the gum—blue stippled line along the gum margin, particularly noted in those with poor oral hygiene. Is rarely seen.
4. Cognitive disability, hyperactive, poor scholastic performance.
5. Peripheral neuropathy—tremors, tingling, numbness, hyperesthesia, wrist drop. The muscle, which are most used are the ones that are affected. Usually, cramps precede the paresis and paralysis.
6. Lead encephalopathy—is an acute emergency. Usually the child manifests with hyperirritability or lethargy and anorexia for 4–6 weeks before the onset of encephalopathy.

There may be the sudden onset of persistent vomiting, ataxia, convulsions, altered consciousness and coma.

Investigations

1. Hemoglobin levels—detect the presence of underlying anemia.

2. Peripheral blood smear—to rule out other causes of anemia. Basophilic stippling is indicative of lead poisoning.
3. Free erythrocyte protoporphyrin and zinc protoporphyrin levels in red blood cells (RBCs)—levels correlate with elevated blood lead levels, especially above 25 μg/dL.
4. Renal function tests (RFTs)—renal tubular dysfunction may occur with very high blood lead levels. RFT is also useful during chelation treatment, especially with potentially nephrotoxic drugs like ethylenediaminetetra-acetic acid (EDTA).
5. Blood lead levels—levels from 10 to 30 μg/dL are usually asymptomatic. Every child showing a single elevated level of 20 μg/dL or 2 levels above 15 μg/dL at least 3 months apart needs to be followed up.
   a. Symptoms usually develop at levels more than 40 μg/dL.
   b. Lead encephalopathy—at levels around 70 μg/dL.
6. X-ray abdomen—shows evidence of lead ingestion. Also acts as an indicator of ongoing lead ingestion in cases, which have increasing lead levels during treatment or for those not responding adequately to treatment.
7. X-ray of long bones—indicated in children with evidence of growth failure. Presence of growth arrest lines (lead lines), is indicative of chronic lead exposure. It occurs at levels above 50 μg/dL.
8. X-ray fluorescence of long bones using radioactive material—for estimation of lead deposits in the long bones. Is not used routinely.

Treatment

1. Chelation therapy is the mainstay of treatment of lead poisoning. Blood lead levels usually fall within 1 week after start of therapy. Rebound increase may occur after stopping the treatment. Monitoring blood lead levels gives an idea of the patient's response to treatment.
2. Causes for persistently elevated blood lead levels:
   a. Hazards in the child's environment persist.
   b. Continued use of contaminated pottery, ceramic, medicines, etc.

c. Bed rest.
d. Immobilization.
e. Acidosis.

3. Chelation involves the binding of the metal by an agent at least two sites, to help excrete it from the body. The ideal chelating agent will bind the lead and increase its excretion from the body. However, the lead-chelate complex may be redistributed to other body tissues.

Dimercaptosuccinic acid (DMSA) is an oral chelating drug, which is the water soluble analog of dimercaprol. DMSA is a four carbon molecule, with two carboxyl and two sulfur groups. The lead molecule binds to the adjoining sulfur and oxygen atoms. The drug reaches a peak concentration after 3–4 hours of oral ingestion. Maximal elimination occurs within 24 hours of administration as a DMSA-cysteine disulfide conjugate. Renal clearance is maximal, with a small amount being excreted in the stools.

Dose: 30 mg/kg/day for 5 days, followed by 20 mg/kg/day for the next 14 days. This will help to decrease the rebound increase in levels that may occur after initial elimination. Blood lead levels give an estimate of the response to treatment, as falling levels indicate elimination from the body.

Side effects of DMSA: Skin rash, pruritus, mucocutaneous lesions, elevated liver enzymes, especially transaminases, which normalize after discontinuation of treatment. Occasional cases of neutropenia have been noted during treatment.

Other Chelating Agents

D-penicillamine: This is a penicillin derivative that is used in chelation of several metals and also in the treatment of Wilson's disease. It is an oral chelating agent, its sulfhydryl group binding to the lead forming a ring compound, which is eliminated.

Penicillamine is rapidly absorbed after oral administration, with peak levels within 1–3 hours after the oral dose. The main route of elimination is the kidneys, with a small amount of fecal elimination. Initial elimination is rapid followed by a sustained elimination of the deeper tissues content of lead.

Dose: 30 mg/kg/day for 1–6 months, given 2 hours before or 3 hours after meal.

Side effects: Related to zinc deficiency like stomatitis, delayed wound healing, desquamations. Also transient leukopenia, thrombocytopenia and abdominal pain are known to occur.

Prognosis

After chelation therapy, there is a definite reduction in the blood lead levels. However, this does not correlate with changes in the symptoms related to elevated lead levels. There is no reversal in the IQ scores, nor in the neurocognitive functions of patients affected by lead poisoning.

However, oral calcium and iron supplements in the diet of these patients will be helpful by decreasing the lead absorption. Oral vitamin C will help in the renal excretion of lead.

Prevention of Lead Poisoning

Prevention of lead poisoning is the cornerstone in the war against lead. Awareness regarding the health hazards and methods to decrease lead exposure will go a long way in reducing toxic exposure.

1. Toddlers between 6 months to 3 years have mouthing behavior and parents must be made aware of the possibility of lead-laden dust particles on the toys.
2. Lead containing paints on toys, ceramic items are sources of danger.
3. Avoid peeling paints in the home.
4. Change lead containing pipes, which supply water laden with lead.
5. Kumkum and other Indian cosmetics like kohl may be sources of lead.
6. Above all, increase the awareness of the toxic effects of lead and the methods of decreasing the exposure and subsequent toxicity.

MERCURY

MERCURY POISONING IN CHILDREN

Mercury is a metal, which has been used for several centuries in various medications. However, long-standing exposure to substances containing this metal are dangerous, as they produce deleterious effects on the various organ systems.

Sources of Mercury

Mercury is found in three forms:

1. Elemental mercury.
2. Inorganic mercury salts.
3. Organic mercury compounds.

Elemental Mercury

Elemental mercury is not absorbed at all, while methylmercury is the most dangerous form of mercury, as almost 90% of the ingested mercury is absorbed from the GIT.

Elemental mercury is present in the liquid form, easily vaporizes and can be inhaled. The vapors are rapidly absorbed into the bloodstream through the alveoli and reach the RBCs can also penetrate into the central nervous system (CNS) and give rise to neurological manifestation. The elemental mercury is not well absorbed from the GIT. Hence, it is mildly toxic when ingested.

Elemental mercury is present in thermometers, sphygmomanometers, etc.

Inorganic Mercury Salts

Inorganic mercury is present in two forms; mercurous (Hg^{+}) or mercuric (Hg^{2+}) forms. Most of the inorganic mercury is present in the mercuric form, especially in batteries and is highly corrosive and toxic. It is absorbed either via oral ingestion or through the skin. It is poorly lipid soluble and accumulates in the kidneys, resulting in renal toxicity. However, due to its slow excretion and the chronic exposure, the mercuric ions can induce the CNS toxicity. These ions are excreted via the feces. Industrial pollution is the common source of inorganic mercury, which is shed into the waterways, like rivers, lakes, etc. Here, it is converted by the aquatic vegetation and organisms into the deadly form of methylmercury, which is ingested by the fish and other live forms. Over 90% is tightly bound to the fish protein and is not destroyed by the cooking methods commonly adopted. Consumption of these marine foods results in slow poisoning with mercury. Mercury can be transferred via the breast milk and also in utero to the developing fetus.

Organic Mercury Compounds

Organic mercury occurs in three forms: Aryl, short-chain alkyl and long-chain alkyl compounds. They are readily absorbed from the GIT, are highly lipid soluble and are corrosive. The aryl and long-chain alkyl mercury compounds are converted to the inorganic form and have toxicity similar to inorganic mercury compounds. Methylmercury is a short-chain alkyl mercury compound, which is rapidly and almost completely absorbed from the GIT and exerts severe toxicity. These compounds have high lipid solubility, cross the blood-brain barrier, placenta and the RBCs. They are distributed in the brain, liver, hair, kidney and skin in a uniform pattern. They can induce neurological symptoms, fetal abnormalities and teratogenic effects.

Exposure to mercury containing products can occur through several routes.

1. Mercury containing disk batteries can cause ulceration of the oral and GIT mucosa.
2. Other batteries can cause hypersalivation and vomiting.
3. Some cosmetics and topical application cream may contain high levels of mercury.
4. Ayurvedic preparations may also contain mercury as an ingredient.
5. Breakage of the newer energy efficient fluorescent bulbs can cause substantial exposure to mercury.

Toxic dose: more than 0.1 μg/kg/day.

Pathophysiology

Methylmercury is the most toxic form of mercury, causing the most severe toxicity in the body, especially in the nervous system. The alkyl mercury is almost completely absorbed from the GIT and undergoes enterohepatic circulation and excreted in the feces. It has a half-life of 65 days.

The Table 5.1 shows some products, which contain mercury and can cause poisoning.

Table 5.1: Products, which contain mercury and can cause poisoning

Elemental	Organic	Inorganic
Thermometers	Antiseptics	Acetaldehyde production
Barometers	Bactericidal	Cosmetics
Batteries	Embalming agents	Disinfectants
Bronzing	Farming industry	Explosives
Calibration instruments	Fungicides	Mercury vapor lamps
Dental amalgams	Germicidal agents	Mirror silvering
Electroplating	Insecticidal products	Perfume industry
Fluorescent lamps	Laundry products	Photography
Mercury lamps	Paper manufacturing	Tattoo inks
Infrared detectors	Wood preservatives	
Jewelry industry		
Manometers		
Neon lamps		
Paints		
Photography		
Silver and gold production		
Semiconductor cells		

Mercury binds to sulfhydryl groups and incapacitates key enzymes involved in the cellular stress response, protein repair and oxidative damage prevention. Methylmercury disrupts the muscarinic cholinergic systems in the brainstem and occipital cortices as well. Methylmercury also inactivates sodium, potassium adenosine triphosphatase (Na^+/K^+ ATPase), which leads to membrane depolarization, calcium entry and eventual cell death. Several pathways may be simultaneously activated converging in apoptosis. Hence, methylmercury also sequesters selenium, hence the enzymes requiring this element are inactivated, causing further damage in the CNS.

Mercury has a direct toxic effect upon the renal tubules resulting in renal tubular necrosis, especially of the proximal tubules.

Inhaled elemental mercury is mostly converted to an inorganic divalent or mercuric form by catalase in the erythrocytes. Elemental mercury as a vapor has the ability to penetrate the CNS, where it is ionized and trapped, attributing to its significant toxic effects. Elemental mercury is not well absorbed by the GIT; therefore, when it is ingested (e.g. thermometers), it is only mildly toxic.

Symptoms

1. Acute mercury poisoning usually presents with cutaneous and neurological symptoms.
2. Inorganic mercury exposure usually presents with vomiting, abdominal pain, hypovolemic shock.
3. Ashen grey mucosa, stomatitis, gingival irritation, loosening of teeth, foul breath.
4. Oliguria and anuria, due to renal tubular necrosis.
5. Inhaled mercury vapors cause fever, chills, shortness of breath.
6. Stomatitis.
7. Lethargy, confusion.
8. Symptoms suggestive of pulmonary embolism can occur following injected mercury.
9. Organic mercury poisoning usually presents with neurological symptoms. Headache, tunnel vision, blurring of vision, dysarthria, ataxia, tremors, hearing disorder, movement disorders, paralysis, mental deterioration.

Signs

No pathognomonic signs of mercury toxicity.

1. Skin changes—cutaneous hyperpigmentation, papulovesicular lesions, erythematous papules especially on palms.
2. Ashen grey lips and mucous membranes.
3. Metal fume fever—manifested by fatigue, weakness, fever, chills, dizziness, headache, abdominal cramping, dyspnea and dysuria.

4. Acrodynia—also known as pink disease and considered to be a mercury allergy; presents with erythema of the palms and soles, edema of the hands and feet, desquamating rash, hair loss, pruritus, diaphoresis, tachycardia, hypertension, photophobia, irritability, anorexia, insomnia, poor muscle tone and constipation or diarrhea; acrodynia does not present in everyone who is exposed to inorganic mercury, but it is an indicator of widespread disease.
5. Erethism—constellation of irritability, excitability, anxiety, insomnia and social withdrawal; erethism is traditionally seen in the chronic phase of the toxicity.
6. Ataxia.
7. Neuropathy—III and VI cranial nerve palsy.
8. Tremulousness.
9. Hearing loss.

Investigations

1. Complete blood count (CBC): Shows extent of anemia, which may be due to GI irritation and blood loss.
2. Serum electrolytes: Hypokalemia, hypophosphatemia.
3. Serum creatinine and blood urea: Impending renal failure.
4. Whole blood mercury level: Usually below 2 μg/dL. Hair samples can also be tested for mercury levels, but is more useful in chronic poisoning with mercury. Usually, levels more than 1.2 μg/dL are indicative of toxicity.
5. Urine levels of mercury: Useful in suspected cases of elemental or inorganic mercury poisoning. Levels above 10–20 μg/dL indicate toxicity. It can also be used to follow the effectiveness of chelation therapy.
6. X-ray abdomen: Elemental mercury is radiopaque and can be visualized in the X-ray. It may be found to outline the intestines. Occasionally, it may also get deposited in the lungs.
7. MRI: It is usually helpful to exclude other causes of CNS symptoms. However, it may be useful in chronic mercury poisoning. Marked atrophy of the calcarine and parietal cortices is noted, along with atrophy of the cerebellar folia. Occasionally, mild frontal atrophy and frontal and subcortical hyperintensities may be noted.

8. Single photon emission computerized tomography—useful for diagnosis in organic mercury toxicity, where it reveals cingulate hypermetabolism.
9. Sural nerve biopsy: It is usually reserved for cases of chronic poisoning. It shows axonal sensorineural neuropathy. Prolonged brainstem evoked potentials may also be noted in chronic cases, especially with organic mercury poisoning.

Treatment

Emergency Management

1. Maintain the airway; ensure that the patient is breathing normally and spontaneously. If any doubts exist about the airway patency, intubate and ventilate the patient.
2. Breathing adequate, administer supplemental oxygen.
3. Maintain adequate circulation and circulatory volume. Administer IV fluids, to counter hypovolemia, as well as maintain the patency of the circulation.
4. Decontamination of the skin: Remove the patient from the exposed area, remove the clothes and wash copiously with water to remove the toxin from the skin.
5. Do not induce emesis. Gastric lavage is indicated if the patient is seen within 4 hours after exposure. In case of organic mercury poisoning and if the mercury is seen in the X-ray, administer activated charcoal, which will adsorb the toxic material. Whole bowel irrigation may also be done, until the rectal effluent is clear. However, its use is doubtful in elemental mercury toxicity.
6. Surgical removal of mercury deposits: From the oral and gingival mucosa, from site of mercury injection, etc. which will help to decrease the toxic effects.
7. Chelation is the treatment of choice.

   Indications for chelation include:

   - Symptomatic patient
   - Likely to develop symptoms
   - High levels of mercury in circulation.

Chelation should be started early in the course of treatment. Mercury binds to the sulfhydryl groups of the cells. The thiol groups in the chelating agents compete with the sulfhydryl groups and bind to the mercury and enhances its excretion from the body.

The 2,3-dimercaptosuccinic acid (DMSA) (succimer), is a chelating agent, which has been found to increase mercury excretion from the body. It is an oral chelator that binds to and increases the urinary elimination of mercury. It has minimal effect on the removal of the other body minerals. Its effect is maximal in the first 8–24 hours after administration. It is relatively safe, though may cause some nausea and GI distress.

Dose: 1 mg/kg every 4 hours for 3 days, followed by a rest period of 4 days. The therapy can be repeated until satisfactory mercury level reduction has taken place in the body.

Other chelating agents available:

a. British anti-Lewisite (BAL): Also known as dimercaprol, it is useful in case of mercury poisoning and in acute poisoning. It is administered IM in a peanut oil base, every 4th hourly. The BAL-mercury complex is dialyzable and the drug can be used in renal failure.

b. D-penicillamine is not used as a first line chelation drug. The drug-mercury complex is eliminated via the urine, hence cannot be administered in cases of renal failure.

8. Hemodialysis: It is used only in case of renal failure, as the renal excretion of the chelator-mercury complex is not adequate. However, by using L-cysteine as a chelator, the hemodialysis may be of use in toxicity reduction.
9. Diet modification: Seafood rich in organic mercury should be avoided completely. Normally the larger fish, the predators like shark, swordfish and tuna have mercury levels above the permissible limits of 1 ppm/million and hence should be avoided. Smaller, herbivorous fish are generally safe to eat.

Minamata Disease

A form of chronic mercury poisoning called Minamata disease, occurred in Japan due to the industrial effluent, which contained inorganic mercury and was allowed to contaminate the water in the bay nearby. The fish converted and stored the organic mercury and in turn the villagers consumed large amounts of the fish, resulting in chronic mercury poisoning manifested as tremors, hearing loss, neurologic deficits and ataxia.

Minamata disease is noted in those who live by the seas and consume large amounts of seafood, especially large fish like tuna, shark, swordfish, etc. These fish concentrate large amounts of methylmercury and hence cause chronic mercury poisoning. The neurological manifestations are severe. Hair, nail and blood levels of mercury are elevated.

Sural nerve biopsy in these patients has shown preferential neuronal loss of the large myelinated nerve fibers.

Most survivors of Minamata disease have chronic neuropathologic conditions, such as the following:

- Ataxia
- Visual field loss
- Psychiatric disturbances
- Sensory loss
- Chronic paresthesias.

Compared with other patients, babies exposed to Minamata disease in utero have more dismal prognosis. Their sequelae include the following:

- Severe developmental delay
- Low birth weight
- Persistent cognitive impairment.

Prevention

1. Safe storage of mercury containing products.
2. Decrease likelihood of mercury spills.
3. Avoid ingestion of fish, which has likely mercury contamination.

Prognosis

The prognosis for mercury poisoning depends on many factors:

1. The chemical form of mercury (inhalation of vapor is worse than inorganic, which may be worse than organic).
2. The dose or amount of mercury poisoning (more leads to poor outcomes or death).

3. Age of person (fetus, neonate and infants more susceptible to lower doses of mercury).
4. Length of exposure (longer exposures result in poor outcomes or death).
5. Route of exposure (inhalation is worst, followed by ingestion and then skin exposure).
6. Person's overall health before exposure (people with pre-existing medical problems do worse than healthy people).

Recovery is usually without sequelae, but pulmonary complications of inhaled toxicity may include interstitial emphysema, pneumatocele, pneumothorax, pneumomediastinum and interstitial fibrosis. Fatal acute respiratory distress syndrome (ARDS) has been reported following elemental mercury inhalation.

ARSENIC

ARSENIC POISONING IN CHILDREN

Arsenic is a heavy metal, long known for its toxicity. It is present everywhere in nature, in plants, seaweeds and in minerals, where it exists in three metallic allotropic forms—alpha or yellow, beta or black and gamma or grey, besides several ionic forms.

Arsenic is used to treat wood, in the form of chromated copper arsenate to make it pest resistant. From these furniture articles, the arsenic can leach out and contaminate the surroundings. It is used in the semiconductor and glass industry. Industrial effluents with arsenic traces can contaminate water bodies, resulting in marine life getting contaminated. Seafoods, especially shellfish are a potent source of contamination. Vegetables, fruits, cereals like rice are also contaminated with arsenic contained in the soil. It is also found in shellfish and seafood as arsenobetaine or 'fish arsenic'. This is the non-toxic form, which is present in trace amounts in all living beings. Arsine gas, which is produced during industrial processes, may be inhaled and can cause severe sudden symptoms of toxicity.

Arsenic has been thought to be linked with the development of Alzheimer's disease. Also, the possibility of its link with gestational diabetes and other precancerous lesions has been suggested. The unborn infant may be at potential risk from arsenic in the water consumed by the pregnant mother.

Arsenic has been used as a medicinal agent for the treatment of promyelocytic leukemias, multiple myeloma, myelodysplastic syndromes and a variety of solid tumors.

Pathophysiology

Arsenic is present in the organic and inorganic forms. The inorganic form is more toxic than the organic form and exists as trivalent and the pentavalent compounds (Fig. 5.2). The trivalent compounds are more toxic than the pentavalent forms. They bind the thiol group and inhibits pyruvate dehydrogenase and several other cellular enzymes, thus limiting, inhibits cellular glucose uptake, gluconeogenesis, fatty acid oxidation and further production of acetyl-CoA; it also blocks the production of glutathione, which prevents cellular oxidative damage. Pentavalent arsenic is

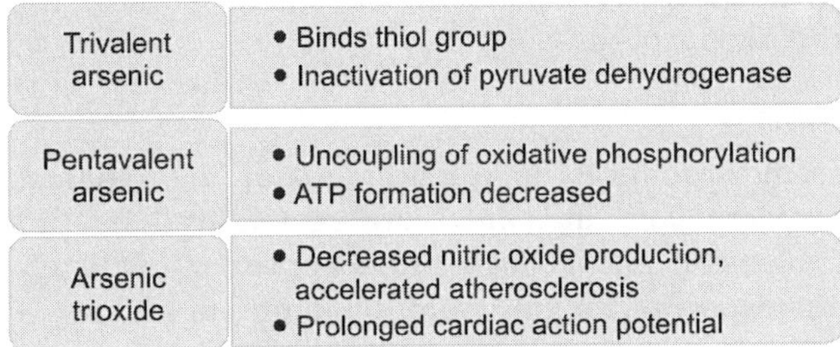

Fig. 5.2: Pathophysiology of action of arsenic

partially converted to the trivalent form, while in its pentavalent form it resembles inorganic phosphate and hence substitutes the phosphate in the glycolytic and cellular respiration pathways. There is uncoupling of the oxidative phosphorylation, with the formation of ADP-arsenate, instead of the high energy ATP molecules. The cells are thus subjected to oxidative stress.

Arsenic also has other actions. Arsenic trioxide has been shown to cause a significant prolongation of cardiac action potential duration at many levels of repolarization producing conduction delay. Electrolyte imbalance appears to enhance this toxicity. The drug appears to inactivate endothelial nitric oxide synthase, leading to a reduction in production and bioavailability of nitric oxide. It also has been associated with inducing/accelerating atherosclerosis, increasing platelet aggregation and reducing fibrinolysis.

Arsine gas produced by the contact of hydrogen with arsenic, causes acute severe toxicity, with severe hemolysis.

The incidence of skin and lung cancers are increased in case of prolonged exposure to arsenic.

Sources of Arsenic

1. Commonly found: As a contaminant in foodstuff like milk, fruit, cereals, seafoods, poultry, rice.
2. Unusual sources: As a rodenticide or herbicide. Transdermal absorption may occur. Also as a contaminant in wine, pigments and glues.
3. Occupational exposure: Semiconductor industry, metal foundry, glass producing industry, etc.

4. Lethal source: Groundwater in shallow wells, used for drinking purposes.

Symptoms

1. Arsenic produces a classical toxidrome, characterized by severe vomiting and diarrhea followed by profound hypotension and collapse. Can appear immediately after acute exposure, ranging from 30 minutes to 4 hours.
2. Characteristic pungent garlic-like smell of the breath.
3. Vomiting, hematemesis, which could be severe.
4. Burning lips, abdominal pain.
5. Intense thirst.
6. Diarrhea, which may be severe cholera like, rice-water stools with dehydration.
7. Passing high-colored urine. This could be indicative of a chronic toxicity with hemoglobinuria and hemolysis.
8. Convulsions.

The stage of acute toxicity lasts 0–4 hours after ingestion and can be fatal. The subacute stage lasts from 24 hours up to 4 weeks after ingestion.

Signs

- Tachycardia, hypotension
- Acute dehydration
- Signs of distress
- White lines called Mees' lines on the nails, resembling traumatic injury
- Shock, acute renal failure
- Peripheral neuropathy resembling Guillain-Barré syndrome, excruciating pain and severe motor weakness
- Cardiac arrhythmias—prolonged QT interval, ventricular fibrillation, etc.
- Altered sensorium
- Seizures
- Coma.

In chronic toxicity, various other signs may be observed.

1. Whitish lines on the fingernails called Mees' lines. Appear like traumatic injuries on the nails.
2. Glove and stocking peripheral neuropathy—symmetric painful paresthesia.
3. Dermatitis, which has a classical appearance of 'dew drops on a dusty road'.
4. Cardiac arrhythmias—prolonged QT interval.
5. Renal and hepatic damage with chronic exposure.
6. Shaking chills and passage of dark urine due to massive hemolytic anemia, usually following exposure to arsine gas.

Investigations

1. CBC—shows microcytic hypochromic anemia. Reticulocyte count to be done to rule out hemolytic anemia.
2. Blood group—to be identified, in case of transfusion requirements.
3. Serum electrolytes—to rule out dyselectrolytemia. Also calcium and magnesium levels in case of convulsions and altered sensorium.
4. Blood arsenic levels—should be below 50 μg/L. In case of toxicity, levels range in hundred to thousands. It is rapidly cleared from the blood, hence is not a very good indicator of toxicity.
5. Urine analysis, urine spot test may show evidence of arsenic. 24-hour urine clearance of inorganic arsenic is the evidence of toxicity. It is the most reliable measurement for acute arsenic toxicity. Levels above 50 μg/24 hours is indicative. However, the levels may drop during the initial 24–48 hours after exposure. It is also essential to differentiate the organic from the inorganic (harmful) metabolites of arsenic, as the total levels could be misleading.
6. Hair and nail levels of arsenic can aid in diagnosis.
7. Serum levels of acetaminophen, to rule out coexistent toxicity.
8. ECG in all leads—for associated cardiac arrhythmias and occasionally cardiac failure.

9. Plain abdominal X-ray—may reveal traces of arsenic in the stomach.
10. Nerve conduction studies—in case of peripheral neuropathy.

Treatment

Emergency Care

1. Maintain and stabilize the airway.
2. Ensure adequate oxygenation and respiration. In case of any alteration in the sensorium, it may be necessary to intubate and ventilate the patient.
3. Rapid volume expansion, to counter the ongoing losses via vomiting or diarrhea. Administer IV fluids rapidly, with continuous blood pressure (BP) monitoring. Massive hemolysis may also require large volume replacement, including repeated blood transfusions.
4. Gastric decontamination is not indicated, unless the patient presents early and there is X-ray evidence of arsenic in the stomach. Orogastric lavage is indicated in acute poisoning, while use of activated charcoal is not indicated, as it does not adsorb arsenic. Whole bowel lavage with polyethylene glycol may be used to prevent GI absorption of arsenic.

Definitive Treatment

1. Chelation is essential for all patients with arsenic poisoning. Chelators bind to the heavy metals and increase its elimination from the body.
   a. Dimercaprol (BAL) is the first-line treatment. It has to be administered intramuscularly, every 4th hourly, mixed in a peanut oil-base. It can be administered safely in patients with renal failure. BAL crosses the blood-brain barrier, hence provides protection against CNS toxicity.
   b. Side effects of BAL include fever, hypertension, worsening of fluid losses, sterile abscesses at injection sites, etc. BAL is contraindicated in G6PD deficiency, as it may cause hemolysis and in those with peanut allergy.
   c. DMSA (succimer) is available as an oral preparation and may be used in arsenic toxicity, though its main use is in the treatment of lead poisoning. Almost all orally

administered DMSA is absorbed and available for chelation, which it does in a 1:1 ratio.

d. Adverse effects of DMSA include nausea, vomiting, elevated transaminases, thrombocytopenia, pruritus and paresthesias.

2. Hemodialysis is indicated when the patient presents with renal failure or massive hemoglobinuria. It has been postulated to be useful in correcting the electrolyte and fluid imbalances associated with renal failure, while the elimination of the arsenic compounds is questionable.
3. Exchange transfusion is indicated in case of exposure to arsine gas, where the RBCs undergo rapid lysis due to the binding and release of toxin, which can cause massive hemolysis.
4. Plasmapheresis—may be considered as a treatment modality in rare cases.

Complications

1. Peripheral neuropathy—which may appear after 2–3 weeks of exposure.
2. Sterile abscess—may develop at the site of injection with BAL.
3. Coma due to recurrent seizures, persistent vomiting, severe dehydration.
4. Bone marrow suppression.
5. Cardiac arrhythmias.
6. Nail changes like Mees' lines.
7. Encephalopathy.
8. Death due to massive hemolysis.

ALUMINIUM PHOSPHIDE

ALUMINIUM PHOSPHIDE TOXICITY IN CHILDREN

Aluminium phosphide is a compound that is an agricultural poison, which is used predominantly to destroy pests and rodents that attack crops and vegetables. It is also used to protect crops during storage and transportation. It is a potent chemical available in the form of tablets and needs to be handled with extreme care.

Toxicity may be direct due to ingestion of the tablets or indirect due to inhalation of the gas released from the degradation of the chemical upon contact with moisture. Dermal absorption of the chemical is rare, unless the skin integrity is broken, wherein the chemical enters the circulation and gives rise to systemic toxicity.

Pathophysiology

After ingestion of the aluminium phosphide tablets, upon contact with the gastric acid, there is release of phosphine gas, which is rapidly absorbed into the systemic circulation. It is transported to the liver and some is absorbed by the lungs, from where most of it is excreted during expiration. The residual portion is converted to phosphate and hypophosphite, which may be excreted in the urine. The phosphine gas is a respiratory poison, which blocks the cytochrome c oxidase enzyme thus inhibiting oxidative phosphorylation, disturbed mitochondrial morphology and altered mitochondrial membrane potential, which causes rapid cell death. Phosphine also inhibits protein synthesis and enzyme activity causing cardiac and pulmonary toxicity. It causes denaturation of the oxyhemoglobin molecule, converting it into methemoglobin. It induces oxidative damage in the brain, lungs and liver. It is postulated that ingestion of aluminium phosphide leads to a high superoxide dismutase activity and low catalase levels that result in formation of a high quantum of free radicals and accelerate lipid peroxidation. The latter, in turn, results in damage to cellular membrane, disruption of ionic barrier, nucleic acid damage and finally cell death.

Symptoms

- Related to the effect of phosphine gas on GIT, kidneys, heart and lungs
- Nausea, vomiting, abdominal pain

- Diarrhea
- Restlessness
- Cough, tightness of the chest
- Cold, clammy skin and extremities
- Tremors, giddiness, lethargy
- Convulsions.

Signs

1. In severe toxicity, the patient has a garlic-like odor in the breath.
2. Cyanosis.
3. Epigastric tenderness.
4. Palpitation, tachycardia.
5. Cold clammy extremities.
6. Tremors, delirium, altered sensorium.
7. Hypotension.
8. Metabolic acidosis.
9. Diffuse bilateral rhonchi.
10. Signs of congestive cardiac failure.
11. Absent ankle reflex.
12. Convulsions.
13. Coma.
14. Delayed effects of phosphide toxicity may be seen after several days, due to the continued absorption of the trace amounts of phosphine gas into the system.

Investigations

1. Serum electrolytes—hypo or hypermagnesemia is a common finding.
2. Acid-base disturbances—metabolic acidosis.
3. Arterial blood gases—to estimate the metabolic acidosis and as a guide to correction and treatment.
4. ECG in all leads—cardiac arrhythmias commonly associated.
5. Chest X-ray—edematous lungs, pleural effusion may be seen.

6. Renal function test (RFT)—to assess the effect of the toxin on the kidneys, as a baseline guide to treatment and to evaluate the prognosis.
7. Ultrasound examination of the abdomen—shows the intestinal congestion, gastric erosions may be visualized.
8. Echocardiogram—to visualize the cardiac function, which may be affected due to aluminium phosphide toxin.
9. Confirmatory tests to detect aluminium phosphide:
   a. Silver nitrate test—using test paper impregnated with silver nitrate, is used to detect the presence of phosphide in gastric fluid. This is a simple and effective test to confirm presence of phosphide in the stomach, which turns the silver nitrate black.
   b. Ammonium molybdate test—using ammonium molybdate reagent in tubes, is used to detect the presence of phosphorus and phosphides in gastric and non-biological tissues suspected to contain aluminium phosphide.
   c. Strip test using dimethyl yellow (0.05%), cresol red (0.1%) and mercuric chloride (1%) in methanol is used for detection of phosphine. The strip turns red in color to indicate the presence of phosphine. This is a highly sensitive test and the reagents have a better shelf-life.
   d. Gas chromatography is a dynamic method to separate and identify the presence of organic compounds in a mixture of inorganic permanent gases.
   e. Electrothermal atomic absorption spectrometry—detects the presence of aluminium in the bone and also in serum.

Treatment

No specific antidote available. Supportive treatment is recommended:

1. Maintain the airway, ensure adequate breathing and administer supplemental oxygen.
2. Maintain IV access and start IV fluids.
3. Gastric lavage, if the patient is brought in early. Administer activated charcoal (1 g/kg body weight) via the lavage to adsorb and inactivate the phosphine.
4. Sodium bicarbonate IV to counter the metabolic acidosis.

5. In case of shock, inotropes may be essential in addition to the IV fluids to maintain the BP.
6. Hemodialysis—in cases of acute renal failure not responding to other supportive measure.

COMPLICATIONS

- Pleural effusion
- Disseminated intravascular coagulation (DIC)
- Arrhythmia
- Acute renal failure
- Hemorrhage
- Pulmonary edema.

Causes of Death

- Massive hemorrhage
- Renal failure
- Cardiac failure
- Respiratory failure
- Intractable seizures
- Pulmonary edema.

SUGGESTED READING

Iron

1. Kleigman RM, Behrman RE, Jenson HB, et al. Nelson Textbook of Pediatrics, 18th edition. Elsevier Health Sciences Division; 2007.
2. Spanierman CS. (2011). Iron toxicity in emergency medicine. www.medscape.com [Accessed May, 2012].

Lead

1. American Academy of Pediatrics Committee on Environmental Health. Lead exposure in children: Prevention, detection and management: Pediatrics. 2006;116:1036-046.
2. Kleigman RM, Behrman RE, Jenson HB, et al. Nelson Textbook of Pediatrics, 18th edition. Elsevier Health Sciences Division; 2007.
3. Pediatric Organ Donation and Transplantation: Policy statement: Organizational principles to guide and define the child health care system and/or improve the health of all children: Commitee on

Hospital Care and Section on Surgery. American Academy of Pediatrics. 2002;109(5):982-84.

Mercury

1. Dean W. DMSA and heavy metal toxicity. www.medscape.com [Accessed May, 2012].
2. Kleigman RM, Behrman RE, Jenson HB, et al. Nelson Textbook of Pediatrics, 18th edition. Elsevier Health Sciences Division; 2007.
3. Olson DA, Ramachandran TS. Mercury toxicity. www.medscape.com [Accessed May, 2012].

Arsenic

1. Baptist DL, Leslie NA. Children playing with poison. Arsenic exposure from CCA treated wood. Journal for Nurse Practitioners. 2008;4(1):48-53.
2. Kleigman RM, Behrman RE, Jenson HB, et al. Nelson Textbook of Pediatrics, 18th edition. Elsevier Health Sciences Division; 2007.
3. Lai MW, Boyer EW, Kleinman ME, et al. Acute arsenic poisoning in two siblings. Pediatrics. 2005;116(1):249-57.
4. Louisiana Department of health and hospitals. Arsenic exposure and toxicity. Information for health care professionals, 2009. www.seet.dhh.la.gov [Accessed December, 2012].
5. Marcus S, Tarabar A. Arsenic toxicity in emergency medicine. www.medscape.com [Accessed August, 2012].

Aluminium Phosphide

1. Bumbrah GS. Phosphide poisoning: A review of literature. Forensic Science International. 2012;214:1-6.
2. Kapoor AK, Sinha US. An epidemiological study of aluminium phosphide poisoning at Allahabad. IIJFMT. 2006;4(1).
3. Suman RL. Pleural effusion a rare complication of aluminium phosphide poisoning. Indian Pediatrics. 1999;36:1161-163.

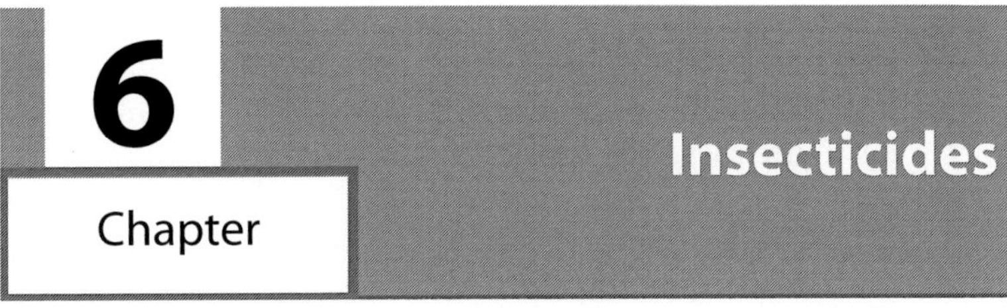

Chapter 6 Insecticides

RODENTICIDE

RODENTICIDE (RAT POISON) TOXICITY

Rodenticides are commonly found household chemicals and one of the most toxic substance that is available in the home. The active ingredients vary, but the commonly used compounds are yellow phosphorus and warfarin-like anticoagulant compounds. As the rodents developed resistance to the warfarin compounds via autosomal dominant gene transmission, long-acting warfarins, called superwarfarins were used and these offer a challenge for treatment modalities. Another compound present in rodenticides is zinc phosphide, which has the smell of rotting fish. Some of the older rodenticides used strychnine, which was derived from a plant source. Thallium and barium may be also components of some rodenticides, though not very widely used these days. Arsenic was another agent that was widely used as a component of rodenticides. Herbal agents, which have some rodenticide activity has been used, containing as the active ingredient, a plant derivative called red squill.

Rodenticide ingestion is usually accidental and hence small quantities are ingested. However, there is also a tendency to lace the intoxicant marijuana with rodenticide to increase its pleasure giving effects. These persons have associated coagulopathies, along with evidence of marijuana intoxication. This has to be kept in mind in cases of adolescent poisonings, where intentional ingestion of rodenticide is a likelihood.

Pathophysiology

1. Based on the chemical component present in the rodenticide, the mechanism of its action is varied.

2. The warfarin group of compounds are divided into two groups: the 4-hydroxycoumarins and the indandiones. Both act by blocking the production of active Vit. K1 via inhibition of K1 reductases. The K1-dependent clotting factors, like II, IV, IX and X, which require Vit. K as a cofactor, cannot be activated in its absence, resulting in coagulopathy involving both extrinsic and intrinsic pathways. The warfarins also increase the capillary permeability throughout the body, predisposing to widespread internal hemorrhage. Lethal hemorrhage may occur after ingestion of even small amounts of superwarfarins, which are more toxic and lethal compared with warfarins. For example, brodifacoum, difenacoum, chlorophacinone, etc.
3. Yellow phosphorus compounds produce chemical burns and damage to the gastrointestinal tract (GIT).
4. Barium acts by moving the potassium intracellularly, thus preventing cellular repolarization. Thallium ingestion results in painful neuropathy.
5. Zinc phosphide is the slowest acting of the commonly used rodenticides and is fairly specific for rodents. It does not affect the other animals that scavenge on the rodents, because the zinc phosphide does not accumulate in the rodent's tissues or muscles. Upon contact of the zinc phosphide with the gastric acids, it releases phosphine gas (PH_3), which damages the RBC membranes and blood vessels causing cardiovascular collapse and GIT irritation. Symptoms appear within 15 minutes to 4 hours after ingestion.
6. Strychnine acts on the nervous system as an antagonist to the neurotransmitter glycine at the postsynaptic spinal cord motor neuron with persistent depolarization.
7. Arsenic combines with the sulfhydryl groups causing blockage of numerous enzymatic reactions and cell signaling pathways.
8. Red squill, a plant derivative, is a cardiac glycoside, resulting in pulmonary edema in the rodents due to glycoside intoxication and the inability of the rodent to vomit. It is not so effective, hence not used commonly these days.

Symptoms

Symptoms depend on the main ingredient in the rodenticide. These may develop after few days after ingestion, due to the long half-life of the main ingredients, by which time, serious damage may have already occurred. May present as:

- Nausea, vomiting, abdominal pain
- Hair loss
- Epistaxis, bleeding gums
- Hematuria with severe flank pain
- Dyspnea, fatigue on exertion
- Bloody diarrhea, melena, extensive ecchymosis
- Seizures
- Hemoptysis
- Excess bleeding or bruising after minor trauma
- Painful neuropathy and hair loss—noted with thallium-containing preparations
- Shortness of breath associated with development of pulmonary edema—with zinc phosphide rodenticides
- Symptoms may prolong for longer durations with the superwarfarins, due to their extended half-life.

Signs

1. Characteristic odor depending on the content of the rodenticide: rotting fish smell due to zinc phosphide.
2. Petechiae and small purpura on the skin and mucous membranes.
3. Bleeding diathesis—hematuria, bloody diarrhea, hemoptysis, bleeding gums, epistaxis, joint bleeds, spontaneous skin bleeds, etc. Occasionally, spontaneous minor bleeds may be noted.
4. Persistent vomiting, melena and electrolyte imbalances.
5. Dyspnea and pulmonary edema.
6. Abdominal pain and intermittent colic.
7. Ataxia, dyspnea, especially with zinc phosphide ingestion.
8. Hypersalivation.
9. Convulsions, coma.

Investigations

1. Complete blood count (CBC)—evidence of hemolysis.
2. Serum electrolytes: to detect any imbalances, especially in cases of persistent vomiting.
3. Blood glucose levels in all patients with altered mental status.
4. Coagulation profile—to assess the coagulation status of the patient.
5. Prothrombin time (PT), partial thromboplastin time (PTT) and international normalized ratio (INR)—precise evaluation of the coagulation status and serves as a guide for further treatment.
6. Serum levels of Vit. K-dependent clotting factors—levels of Vit. K-dependent factors, II, VII, IX and X are decreased, while other coagulation factor levels are normal.
7. Serum acetaminophen level—to rule out coingestion.
8. X-ray abdomen—some rodenticides contain heavy metals like thallium, barium, arsenic, etc. which are radiopaque.

Treatment

1. Try to obtain the container, so that the specific product can be noted and its contents ascertained accurately.
2. Decontaminate the patient. Move the patient from the site, remove the clothes and wash the exposed parts of the body to remove all traces of the rodenticide.
3. Secure the airway and in case of altered mental status, intubate the patient. Severe respiratory compromise with zinc phosphide is also an indication for intubation.
4. Secure the IV line to maintain the IV access.
5. Gastric decontamination—in case the patient presents early to the hospital or in cases of massive overdose. Insert the orogastric tube and administer to the stomach, wash with activated charcoal, which will adsorb the chemical and prevent further intestinal absorption.
6. In case of seizures, administer benzodiazepines to abort the seizure activity.
7. In case of active bleeding and documented coagulopathy, administer Inj. Vit. K. Treatment may be initiated with INR

levels greater than 2. In case of frank bleeding, it may be essential to correct the coagulopathy by administering fresh frozen plasma, which may need to be repeated depending on the patient's response. In case there is no active bleed nor evidence of coagulopathy, there is no need to administer prophylactic Vit. K, as this may mask the onset of the coagulopathy.

Dose of Vit. K to be administered intramuscularly. Based on the severity of bleeding (American College of Chest Physicians):

a. Serious bleeding: 10 mg.
b. Non-serious bleeding:
   - INR 6 to 10: 0.5 to 1 mg
   - INR 10 to 20: 3 to 5 mg
   - INR > 20: 10 mg.

Continue treatment until the PT normalizes and repeat the INR after 24–48 hours, to ensure normalization.

8. In case of poisoning with the superwarfarins, the coagulopathy may persist for a longer duration of treatment and repeated doses of Vit. K may be required to correct the coagulation profile.
9. Occasionally, the zinc phosphide containing products release phosphine gas, which can result in severe hemolysis. This severe condition may be an indication for exchange transfusion.
10. In case of severe bleeding such as GI bleeding or intracerebral hemorrhage—fresh frozen plasma transfusion may be required.
11. In case of renal failure, hemodialysis may be indicated.

Complications

1. Severe hematuria.
2. Hematemesis.
3. Spontaneous intra-abdominal hemorrhage.
4. Intracerebral hemorrhage.
5. Intractable seizures.
6. Spontaneous hemoperitoneum.
7. Death.

Follow-up

It is essential in cases of toxicity with rodenticides of superwarfarin groups, due to the delayed onset of action. It is essential to follow-up these children, until the INR returns to normal and all the coagulation parameters are normalized.

Prognosis

Ingestion of superwarfarin constitutes the majority of the rodenticide exposures. However, the outcomes are usually benign due to the low amount of rodenticide consumed and early medical care. Herbal red squill-containing compounds usually produce only GIT symptoms and are easy to treat and recovery is complete. Poisoning with metals like thallium and arsenic-containing compounds may produce long-term sequelae like neuropathy, especially peripheral and the prognosis in these cases is guarded. Zinc phosphide toxicity could cause a higher mortality rate as compared to the other agents.

Prevention

1. Ensure that all poisons are kept in the original containers and nothing is left lying loose outside.
2. Ensure that the rodenticide mixed with food is not placed at locations easily accessible to small children.
3. After use, close the containers tightly and place them out of reach from small children.

ORGANOPHOSPHORUS COMPOUNDS

ORGANOPHOSPHORUS POISONING

Organophosphorus compounds are found in insecticides and pesticides, which are commonly used around the home as insect killers and repellents.

The active ingredient is organic phosphate, the concentration of which varies from 1% to 95%. The toxicity of the compound varies, depending on the concentration of the active ingredient. Absorption occurs from all routes—ingestion, inhalation, absorption.

Pathophysiology

Organophosphates are cholinesterase inhibitors. They form an initially reversible bond with the enzyme cholinesterase.

Acetylcholine (ACh) is the neurotransmitter released at all postganglionic parasympathetic nerve endings and at the synapses of both sympathetic and parasympathetic ganglia. It is also released at the skeletal muscle myoneural junction and serves as a neurotransmitter in the central nervous system.

Cholinesterase is present in the cell in two forms—true cholinesterase, which is present in the tissues and erythrocytes and pseudocholinesterase, which is present in the tissues and liver. True cholinesterase rapidly hydrolyses acetylcholine that is present in the nerve endings of the sympathetic and parasympathetic nerve endings and skeletal muscle receptors. This action occurs rapidly after exposure. Once the enzyme is inactivated, there is accumulation of acetylcholine at the muscarinic and nicotinic receptors of the neurons and subsequently disrupts the nerve transmission in both the central and peripheral nervous system.

Symptoms and signs depends on the extent and route of poisoning. Symptoms may be seen within 30 minutes up to 3 hours after exposure. Normally, a history of accidental exposure is forthcoming. Patients may present with vomiting, abdominal pain, diarrhea, while some may be brought unconscious to the emergency room. The signs are usually secondary to the agent, the route of exposure and the quantity of exposure. A high index of suspicion is essential to make a diagnosis of organophosphorus poisoning, so that early treatment can be instituted.

Symptoms of Toxicity

Symptoms start within 30 minutes to 3 hours after exposure. Symptoms depend on the route of exposure. Blurred vision, headaches, giddiness and weakness are the common central nervous system (CNS) symptoms. Abdominal pain, inability to control urine output may also be presenting symptoms.

The earliest symptoms occur following inhaled toxins. Symptoms based on the system involvement as mentioned in Table 6.1.

Table 6.1: Symptoms and signs of organophosphorus poisoning

Muscarinic receptors	Nicotinic receptors	Central receptors
Cardiovascular	**Cardiovascular**	**General effects**
Bradycardia	Tachycardia	Anxiety
Hypotension	Hypertension	Restlessness
Respiratory	**Musculoskeletal**	Dysarthria
Rhinorrhea	Weakness	Tremors
Bronchorrhea	Fasciculations	Convulsions
Bronchospasm	Cramps	Ataxia
Cough	Paralysis	Insomnia
Gastrointestinal		Absent reflexes
Abdominal cramps		Circulatory collapse
Nausea/vomiting		Respiratory depression
Increased salivation		Coma
Diarrhea		
Fecal incontinence		
Eyes		
Blurred vision		
Increased lacrimation		
Miosis		
Genitourinary		
Urinary incontinence		
Glands		
Excessive salivation		

Important symptoms 'dumbels', which could indicate organophosphate poisoning, as shown in Figure 6.1. A high index of suspicion of poisoning is essential to make a diagnosis, which is very essential to start early treatment, which in turn affects the patient's recovery.

Pathogenesis of Symptoms

The symptoms depend on the system involved. There is no definite pattern for the systemic involvement, hence the varied methods of presentation. A high index of suspicion is essential for arriving at the accurate diagnosis (Box 6.1).

Diagnosis

1. Clinical symptoms and signs.
2. Serum cholinesterase levels—reduction in serum levels correlates with organophosphorus poisoning.
   - Mild poisoning—levels ranging from 20% to 50% of normal activity
   - Moderate poisoning—from 10% to 20% of normal activity
   - Severe poisoning—less than 10% of normal activity.
3. Serum pseudocholinesterase levels—decreased in cases of organophosphate poisonings.
4. Electrocardiogram (ECG)—shows evidence of cardiac involvement. Prolonged QTc interval, elevated ST segment, inverted T waves, prolonged PR interval.
5. Demonstration of p-nitrophenol levels by gas chromatography or by thin layer chromatography.
6. Therapeutic trial—with atropine and PAM. Initial rapid improvement is seen in the patient's condition.

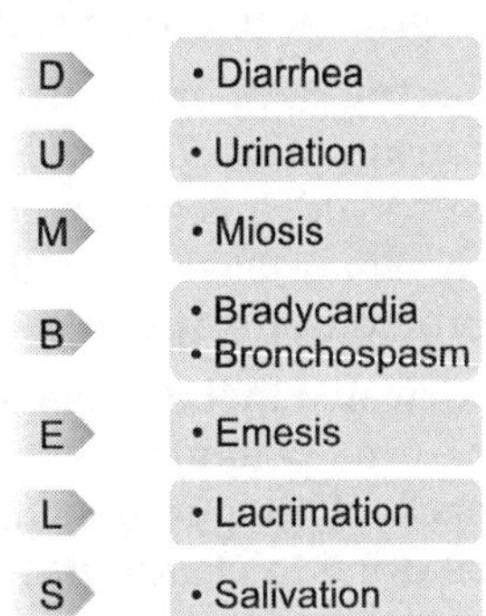

Fig. 6.1: Important symptoms of organophosphorus poisoning

Treatment

1. Immediate treatment—decontamination of the patient.

Box 6.1: Pathogenesis of symptoms

Respiratory

- Muscarinic: Bronchorrhea, bronchospasm, laryngospasm
- Nicotinic: Weakness, respiratory and oropharyngeal muscle paralysis

Neurological

- Type I paralysis: Persistent depolarization due to muscarinic and nicotinic receptors
- Type II paralysis: Intermediate, 4–18 day later; neck flexor and proximal limb weakness
- Type III paralysis: 2–4 week late; distal weakness, ataxia, fasciculation, inhibitory paralysis

Gastrointestinal

- Muscanic: Similar to gastroenteritis—diarrhea, vomiting, abdominal cramps

Cardiac

- Direct myocardial toxicity
- Nicotinic and cholinergic activity: Hemodynamic alterations

a. Remove the patient from the site of exposure.
b. Change the clothes.
c. Wash the skin with plenty of soap and water to prevent further absorption of the poison from the skin.
d. Medical staff to be protected with gloves, eyewear and gowns before decontamination procedures.

2. Gastric emptying—to be done if patient arrives within 1 hour of consumption. Gastric lavage is the preferred mode, compared to forced emesis, which can precipitate seizures. Activated charcoal, 0.5–1 g/kg to be instilled after gastric lavage, to promote adsorption of the poison from the stomach.
3. Airway—to be secured and maintained. Place patient in neutral position to maintain open airway, prevent falling back of tongue and airway obstruction. Throat suction to be done to clear out the secretions. Intubate and ventilate if sensorium is altered or likely to deteriorate.
4. Ensure breathing and adequate air exchange. Administer supplemental oxygen.

5. Maintenance of circulation—intravenous (IV) fluids to be administered to maintain the circulatory volume. Usually isotonic saline or Ringer lactate needs to be administered, depending on the volume depletion and patient's general condition.
6. Specific antidote therapy.

Specific Antidote Therapy

Anticholinergics

Atropine: This is the specific antidote against the organophosphorus poisons. However, atropinization must be instituted only after the supportive measures have been undertaken and the patient is adequately stabilized.

Atropine is administered in the dosage of 0.03–0.04 mg/kg/dose IV to be given stat, else 2 mg IV bolus dose can be given. The same dose is repeated every 10–15 minutes, until adequate atropinization is achieved. Usually 5–6 doses are adequate to produce atropinization, but this again depends on the severity of toxicity.

Indicators of atropinization—flushed skin, dry mouth, moderately dilated pupil, tachycardia, heart rate greater than 140/min, decreased secretions, reduced bowel sounds.

Once the atropinization is achieved, continue administration of atropine at a maintenance dose of 0.02–0.08 mg/kg/h, to ensure that the patient is satisfactorily atropinized. Maximal dosing is usually required on day 1 and tends to decrease over the next few days. However, atropine does not reverse the skeletal muscle effects of organophosphorus.

Cholinesterase reactivator

Pralidoxime (PAM, pralidoxime 2 aldoxime chloride)—this is used to reactivate the phosphorylated cholinesterase by binding to the organophosphorus molecule. PAM acts by:

1. Converting the organophosphate into an inactive and harmless molecule.
2. Protecting the enzyme from further deactivation—this is a transient action.
3. The inhibited alkyl phosphorylated enzyme is reactivated, so that the active unit can be freed.

Pralidoxime (PAM) is used to reverse the nicotinic effects at the skeletal neuromuscular junction. PAM gives best results, if administered early during treatment to prevent complete binding of acetylcholinesterase. Once this has occurred, the recovery will be slower, as receptor regeneration has to occur, before recovery occur.

Dosage of PAM: 25–50 mg/kg slow IV dissolved in 5% dextrose saline over 20 minutes. Can be repeated after 1 hour, if muscle weakness persists. PAM needs to be administered every 12th hourly.

Patient begins to show improvement within 10–40 minutes after administration of PAM. Effective plasma concentration is 4 mg/L.

Side effects of PAM:

- Nausea
- Muscle weakness
- Tachycardia
- Drowsiness
- Visual disturbances.

Continuous monitoring is the key to good prognosis in cases of organophosphorus poisoning.

Prognosis

Outcome depends on the early administration of adequate treatment. Benign outcomes can be anticipated in most cases, as the amount ingested is small in most cases.

PYRETHRUM INSECTICIDE

PYRETHRUM TOXICITY IN CHILDREN

Pyrethrum is the general name, which refers to two groups of insecticides—the pyrethrins and the pyrethroids. Pyrethrins are natural insecticides that are extracted from the flower of the *Chrysanthemum* plant. The flowers are dried and powdered to extract the oils in them, which contains almost 30% of pyrethrin as the active ingredient. Pyrethrin I and II are the commonly used compounds.

The synthetic and semisynthetic derivatives of the chrysanthemic acid compounds are called pyrethroids. The pyrethroids are more effective than the naturally derived pyrethrins and last longer in the environment. Pyrethroids are of two types—type I (allethrin) and type II (deltamethrin and fenvalerate).

Pyrethrins are present in insecticides used in agriculture, antilice preparations, as well as insect repellants. It is also used in the grain storage barns, as well as in poultry pens to control the pests. The pyrethroids, especially allethrin is present in the commonly used mosquito coils. Pyrethroids are also present in antiscabies preparations, pet sprays and shampoos.

Both the pyrethrins and pyrethroids are usually mixed with solvents or carriers to produce the commercial grade products. These may be inert substances, which increase the toxicity of the final chemical product.

Mode of Action

Natural pyrethrins are contact poisons, which penetrate the nervous system of the insect and can knock it down upon contact with the chemical. However, the pyrethrins are rapidly detoxified by the insect's enzymes, which can result in only temporary immobility and recovery of the pest. Pyrethrins are destroyed rapidly by natural sunlight and are only slightly water soluble. They are extremely toxic to aquatic life, hence is usually not sprayed into water.

Pyrethroids are commonly used in synthetic insecticides, which are sprayed on crops, to control flying insects, etc. They are also rapidly degraded by natural sunlight, while rain or snow remove the compounds from the air. The compounds bind strongly to the soil and are eventually degraded by the microorganisms in the soil. However, the insecticides may be sprayed on to the plants and thus, may be found on the leaves, fruits and vegetables. The compound allethrin is present in the commonly used mosquito repellent coils together with another chemical called N-N-diethyl-meta-toluamide (DEET), which facilitates the entry of the permethrin into the skin.

Routes of Exposure

Pyrethrum toxicity can occur by different routes:

1. Dermal exposure of the sprayed insecticide.
2. Dermal absorption of the applied insecticide.
3. Inhalation of the sprayed insecticide.
4. Ingestion of the insecticide residues present on the fruits and vegetables.
5. Accidental ingestion of insecticides, mosquito coils, etc.

Infants and children are more likely to develop toxicity with smaller doses following dermal exposure.

Pathophysiology

Upon exposure to the pyrethrum compounds, the chemical enters the body and is rapidly metabolized in the liver by ester hydrolysis and hydroxylation to inactive acids and alcohol components. These metabolites are less toxic than the parent compound. These metabolites are excreted in the urine and feces and are usually neither stored in the body nor excreted in the human milk. However, pyrethrin I and II are excreted unchanged in the feces. If exposure is high or prolonged, the compounds can accumulate in the fatty tissues in the body and occasionally, it is stored in the hair and skin also.

All the pyrethroid derivatives act on the CNS to cause various symptoms and signs. Allethrin is a type I pyrethroid, which lacks the cyano group and act on the sodium channels, causes repetitive discharges in the nerve fibers with resultant hyperexcitation of the nerves. There may also be some alterations in the calcium channels, which aggravate the symptoms caused by type I pyrethroids. The type II pyrethroids act by nerve membrane depolarization and nerve block.

Permissible daily dose of permethrin (according to WHO and UN Food and Agriculture Organization): 3 mg/day for adults. Pediatric dose is not specified.

Symptoms

1. Depends on the route of absorption.
2. Itching, burning, stinging, feeling of warmth—upon skin contact with pyrethroids.
3. Dizziness, nausea, headache—on exposure to small amounts.
4. Muscle twitching.
5. Loss of awareness.
6. Convulsions.

Signs

1. Skin rash, erythema, tingling sensation.
2. Flushing, facial swelling.
3. Nasal stuffiness, headache.
4. Difficulty in breathing, dyspnea, asthmatic breathing.
5. Tremors.
6. Ataxia, incoordination of movements and gait.
7. Convulsions.
8. Altered sensorium.
9. Behavioral alterations—violent behavior.

Signs of chronic toxicity may occasionally occur and are related to absorption of pyrethrum via the lungs. It can cause allergic reactions, producing itching, pricking and local burning sensations, which can last within a few days.

Investigations

1. CBC—to rule out infections.
2. Serum electrolytes—in cases of severe toxicity, where the patient presents in altered sensorium. Also essential in cases of dehydration due to persistent vomiting and nausea after ingestion.
3. Serum glucose—in case of persistent seizures, in altered sensorium, persistent vomiting.

4. Gastric lavage fluid—for toxicology screen. It is useful, if the patient is seen soon after consumption of the toxic substance.
5. Patch testing for the pyrethrum compounds, in case of dermal contact. The test may not be easily available in all laboratories.
6. Computerized tomography (CT) scan and magnetic resonance imaging (MRI) of brain in case of convulsions without known cause or if patient is in altered sensorium.

Treatment

There is no specific antidote for pyrethroids. Treatment is only supportive care, which are as follows:

1. Maintain airway, ensure adequate breathing, provide supplemental oxygen.
2. Intravenous (IV) access to be established and administer IV fluids. In case of dehydration, fluids need to be administer rapidly.
3. Administer diazepam or lorazepam in case the patient has convulsions. It is essential to abort the seizure at the earliest. Sometimes, patients may have recurrent seizures, hence long-acting anticonvulsants may be needed.
4. Gastric lavage may be useful in case the patient presents to the hospital early, after consumption of the toxic substance. Pyrethroids are not readily absorbed from the stomach, however, their presence may help in establishing the diagnosis and decrease to passage into the intestines.

Prognosis

Most cases of acute pyrethroid poisoning recover within 1–6 days with normal neurological function. Sometimes, in cases of persistent seizures, the fatality rates may range from 12.5% to 25%, as has been shown in reports from India.

SUGGESTED READING

Rodenticide

1. Fishel F. Pesticide poisoning symptoms and first aid. www.extension.missouri.edu/publications/DisplayPub.aspx?P=G1915 [Accessed January, 2013].

2. Iowa Statewide Poison Control Center. Long-acting anticoagulant rodenticides. www.iowapoison.com [Accessed December, 2012].
3. Kliegman RM, Behrman RE, Jenson HB, et al. Nelson Textbook of Pediatrics, 18th edition. Elsevier Health Sciences Division; 2007.
4. Lung D, Tarabar A. Rodenticide toxicity. Updated 2011. www.medscape.com [Accessed December, 2012].
5. Minnesota Poison Control System, Hennepin County Medical Center. www.michigan.gov [Accessed December, 2012].
6. University of Kansas Hospital Poison Control Center. www.kumed.com [Accessed December, 2012].

Organophosphorus Compounds

1. Joshi S, Biswas B. Management of organophosphorus poisoning. Update in Anaesthesia. 2005;19:1-2. www.nda.ox.ac.uk/wfsa/html/u19/u19130.1.htm [Accessed December, 2012].
2. Kliegman RM, Behrman RE, Jenson HB, et al. Nelson Textbook of Pediatrics, 18th edition. Elsevier Health Sciences Division; 2007.

Pyrethrum Insecticide

1. Agency for toxic substances and disease registry. Toxic substances portal. Public health statement for pyrethrins and pyrethroids. Updated September 2003. www.atsdr.cdc.gov/phs/phs.asp?id=785&tid=153 [Accessed December, 2012].
2. Garg P. Mosquito coil (Allethrin) poisoning in two brothers. Indian Pediatrics. 2004;41:1177-178.
3. Pyrethrins and Pyrethroids. http://extoxnet. orst.edu/pips/pyrethri.htm [Accessed December, 2012].

7 Chapter Gases

CAMPHOR POISONING

CAMPHOR POISONING IN CHILDREN

Camphor was obtained by distillation of the bark of the *Cinnamomum camphora.* However, these days it is produced commercially from turpentine oil. Camphor is available in various forms such as granules, crystals, blocks or camphorated oil. It has a penetrating pungent odor with an aromatic taste. It is used as karpoora in the Indian households, which is essential for religious worship, as well as used for flavoring in foods. The camphorated oil is used as a muscle relaxant and for treatment of cold, headache, joint pain, cardiac and central nervous system stimulant. The camphor oil could be mistakenly consumed instead of castor oil and the granules and crystals can be easily placed in the oral cavity following which they rapidly disintegrate.

Toxic dose: greater than 20 mg/kg or greater than 500 mg, whichever is greater.

Regular use of camphor containing products can result in a cumulative effect resulting in chronic toxicity.

Symptoms

Symptoms can occur immediately after exposure to camphor.

- Nausea and vomiting
- Lethargy
- Convulsions
- Coma.

Signs

- Characteristic odor of camphor from the patient
- Hyperactivity
- Lethargy
- Tenderness in epigastric region
- Dehydration from persistent vomiting
- Convulsions within 90 minutes of ingestion
- Muscle fasciculation
- Respiratory depression
- Coma.

Investigations

No specific tests are needed, when the diagnosis is obvious.

- Complete blood count (CBC) will show leukocytosis
- Serum levels of camphor, may show elevated levels
- Urine toxin scan—to rule out associated toxicities
- Chest X-ray will show any evidence of associated respiratory infection, for which the camphor containing formulation may have been used.

Treatment

No specific antidote.

Supportive Treatment

1. Do not induce vomiting.
2. Local irrigation of the skin, in case of dermal application of camphor containing medications. Remove clothing and wash with plenty of water.
3. Local irrigation of the eyes, in case of splash injury.
4. Gastric decontamination to be done in case the patient presents within 1 hour of ingestion and if the patient is conscious and alert. Administer activated charcoal in the dose of 1 g/kg, which will help to adsorb the ingested toxin.
5. Observe the patient for 4 hours. If asymptomatic after 4 hours, the patient can be discharged and sent home.

6. In case patient is symptomatic, treat accordingly.
7. In case of convulsions, administer benzodiazepines, preferably IV medication, so as to abort the convulsion rapidly.
8. In case of dehydration, administer IV fluids.
9. Observe the patient for changes in sensorium.

Counseling

In case of accidental poisoning, the parents need to be counseled regarding the potential toxicity of camphor and to avoid placement of the products in easy to reach locations.

Preparations Containing Camphor as an Ingredient

1. Vicks VapoRub cream and ointment.
2. Heet liniment.
3. Bengay ointment.
4. Mentholatum ointment.
5. Campho-phenique ointment.

CARBON MONOXIDE

CARBON MONOXIDE POISONING IN CHILDREN

Carbon monoxide (CO) is a colorless, odorless and tasteless, but highly toxic gas. It is produced from the incomplete combustion of the organic matter, especially the incomplete burning of fossil fuels, gasoline, etc. CO poisoning is usually unintentional and occurs, when the vehicle ignitions are left running for long duration and the fumes can build up especially in confined spaces. It can also result from forest fires, fumes from improperly maintained appliances such as generators and other fuel consuming appliances, burning wood or charcoal, stoves, lanterns or heating systems. The winter season is the time when the CO poisoning is more likely due to the need for usage of heating apparatus and systems.

Methylene chloride is a volatile liquid used in paint removers, solvents degreasers, etc. The vapors of this liquid are generally exhaled, but up to 20% can be stored in the tissues and released slowly. It is metabolized into CO and slowly released into the circulation causing prolonged exposure and toxicity, which could last more than double the time that caused by direct exposure to CO fumes. Cigarette smoking also increases the susceptibility to CO poisoning, as the baseline carboxyhemoglobin levels are already elevated in the smokers.

Pathophysiology

Following exposure to CO fumes, there occurs a combination of tissue hypoxia plus the inflammatory response.

The CO readily crosses the capillary membranes in the lungs. It has a great affinity to the heme moiety of hemoglobin and binds to it avidly. The oxygen can only bind to that amount of hemoglobin that is proportional to the partial pressure of oxygen in the respired air. The carboxyhemoglobin complex shifts the oxygen dissociation curve to the left, with resultant inability of oxygen to be released into the tissues and hypoxia ensues (Fig. 7.1).

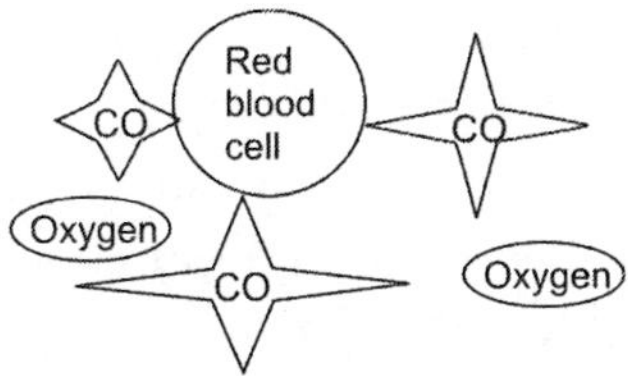

Fig. 7.1: Site of action of carbon monoxide

Carbon monoxide also directly binds the extracellular proteins like myoglobin, cytochromes and the enzymes like nitric oxide synthase and guanylate cyclase. The oxygen binding sites are further decreased thus worsening the hypoxia.

Carbon monoxide binding to mitochondrial cytochrome results in disruption of the mitochondrial electron transport chain. The oxidative phosphorylation process is incomplete, producing oxygen free radicals instead of the energy adenosine triphosphate (ATP) molecules. Thus, there is a hypoxic effect together with oxidative stress that interferes with the body functions.

Due to the reactive oxygen released, there are inflammatory changes that occur, especially in the brain causing lipid peroxidation, which alters the myelin basic protein that leads to autoimmune activity against the cerebral protein. There is also a systemic inflammatory response syndrome occurring against the other body tissues.

Symptoms

- Usually vague, hence can be easily misdiagnosed
- Symptoms similar to a viral infection can be the presenting features
- Headache and dizziness
- Nausea and vomiting
- Difficulty and shortness of breath
- Loss of muscle control
- Loss of consciousness
- Hyperventilation attack
- Non-specific symptoms.

Signs

May be non-specific.

- Evidence of exposure to fumes like burnt hair and singed skin
- Cherry-red coloration of skin is classical of carboxyhemoglobin formation
- Cyanotic, pale and mottled skin
- Hypoxia and hypotension

- Tachypnea
- Tachycardia
- Hyperthermia
- Occasionally, hypertension may occur
- Rales may be heard due to non-cardiogenic pulmonary edema
- Ophthalmic examination reveals bright red retinal veins is an early sign of CO toxicity
- Loss of consciousness with abnormally low Glasgow Coma Scale.

Late signs are memory disturbance, amnesia, lethargy, stupor, coma, gait and vestibular dysfunction, rigidity, emotional lability and impaired judgement and cognitive functions may be seen.

Investigations

1. Complete blood count (CBC)—to note the hemoglobin level. Anemia may be noted.
2. CO oximetry—to detect the presence of carboxyhemoglobin (COHb). It is elevated in CO exposure.
3. Blood gas analysis—venous samples are used to measure the levels of COHb by spectrophotometric method.
4. Arterial blood gases—to detect elevated lactate levels, which may reveal acid-base deficit. Duration of exposure and amount of cellular hypoxia are indicated by the base deficit.
5. Urinalysis—may show evidence of rhabdomyolysis as evidenced by hemoglobinuria.
6. Coagulation parameters—to rule out disseminated intravascular coagulation (DIC) and multiple organ dysfunction syndrome (MODS).
7. Cardiac enzymes to be measured when patient has complaints of chest pain or has CO exposure for longer duration.
8. In case of altered mental status, measure serum ethanol levels and toxicology screen, if possible.
9. X-ray of the chest to be done, when the patient complains of breathing difficulty. The presence of X-ray findings such as haziness, ground-glass appearance or intra-alveolar edema indicate a poor prognosis.

10. Computed tomography (CT) scan of the brain when the patient is in altered sensorium, may show hypodense areas in the globus pallidus and white matter, which is an early finding in CO toxicity. Changes, if noted are predictive of subsequent neurological complications.
11. Electrocardiogram (ECG)—ischemia, arrhythmias secondary to hypoxia may be noted. ECG needs to be performed in all patients, although it may be normal, despite myocardial injury due to toxicity. Moderate to severe toxicity is generally associated with myocardial damage.

Treatment

1. Immediately remove the patient from the source of exposure.
2. Keep the patient calm, as the agitation increases the oxygen demand.
3. Supply oxygen using a non-rebreather mask. Provide high flow oxygen.
4. Maintain the airway. If patient is comatose, need to intubate and ventilate immediately.
5. Start cardiac monitoring and perform the ECG in all 12 leads.
6. Assessment of COHb by venous or arterial blood gas analysis, gives an idea of the extent of COHb concentration, hypoxia and also gives an estimation of the amount of oxygen therapy needed as treatment. The half-life of COHb is 5 hours 30 minutes, while breathing room air and decreases 30–90 minutes with 100% oxygen and is down to 15–23 minutes at 2.5–2.8 atm of 100% oxygen. This can be used as a guide for treatment with hyperbaric oxygen.
7. Hyperbaric oxygen treatment is used in moderate to severe CO poisoning in patients with severe hypoxia, neurological symptoms, refractory acidosis and myocardial dysfunction.

Complications

1. Acute respiratory distress syndrome.
2. Disseminated intravascular coagulation.
3. Acute tubular necrosis.

4. Multiple organ dysfunction syndrome.
5. Leukoencephalopathy of subcortical white matter. Late signs may develop within 1 month of exposure.

Criteria for Discharge

- COHb less than 10%—discharge after observation
- Mild symptoms—treat with 100% oxygen and discharge after 4 hours
- Levels above 15% need in patient care
- Re-evaluate after 24–48 hours for delayed symptoms.

HYDROGEN SULFIDE

HYDROGEN SULFIDE TOXICITY IN CHILDREN

Hydrogen sulfide is a colorless gas having a distinct odor of rotten eggs. The gas is produced in nature from bovine excreta. But the major route of toxicity is the industrial production of hydrogen sulfide (H_2S) gas. It is a byproduct in the refinery of natural and refinery gas, paper production and carbon dioxide production.

Children are more prone to the toxicity of this gas, as they spend considerably more time outdoors than adults. Also they are intensely active, while outdoors, with resultant higher respiratory rates, hence more gas inhalation. The developing lungs are brain are more susceptible to toxicity, with permanent damage occurring due to repeated or continuous low dose exposure. Sudden exposure to high doses can be fatal with even one or two breaths, the so called 'slaughterhouse sledgehammer' effect.

Pathophysiology

Since H_2S is a gas, its toxic effects are observed following the inhalation of the gas. The fumes are pungent and cause irritation of the respiratory tract. The H_2S is easily absorbed into the tissues as it has a very high lipid solubility. It is attracted to the ferric moiety of hemoglobin and causes inhibition of cytochrome oxidase enzyme. Aerobic respiration is thus inhibited, with results comparable to cyanide toxicity in the body. All body organs are affected, especially the central nervous system (CNS) and the respiratory tracts and the severity of the symptoms depends on the extent of exposure. Low levels of the gas exposure causes local symptoms of irritation of the eyes and mucosa. High levels of exposure can result in sudden death due to the involvement of the brainstem and cardiorespiratory arrest.

Toxic Dose Greater than 700 ppm

Although the gas has a typical smell of rotten eggs, at higher concentrations the olfactory glands are overwhelmed, hence the subject is not aware of being exposed to toxic levels of this gas. Toxicity could result from low dose exposure, sudden high level exposure or very high level exposure. The symptoms vary depending on the type and amount of gas inhaled.

Symptoms

Headache, asthenia—common with low level exposure and with high level exposure, the following symptoms are common:

- Cough and dyspnea
- Nausea and vomiting
- Confusion and vertigo
- Possible loss of consciousness
- Hemoptysis
- Exposure to very high level, may result in cardiorespiratory arrest from brainstem involvement
- Sudden loss of consciousness (knockdown effect)
- Seizures
- Myocardial infarction.

Signs

- Hydrogen sulfide is an irritant gas, causing signs of irritation even at low doses
- Conjunctivitis, at low levels of exposure
- Pharyngitis
- Colored line on the gingival margin (grey-green)
- With high level exposure, the signs vary
- Bradycardia
- Dizziness and impaired memory
- Tremulousness, agitation
- Keratoconjunctivitis, blepharospasm, corneal ulceration
- Cyanosis
- Wheezing and difficulty in breathing
- Disequilibrium
- Olfactory paralysis
- Respiratory arrest.

Investigations

1. Oxygen tension, pO_2 and calculated oxygen saturation within normal range, unless there is concomitant pulmonary edema.

2. Metabolic acidosis.
3. Arterial blood gas (ABG) shows evidence of metabolic acidosis.
4. Venous blood gas measurement shows abnormally high oxygen tension, due to decreased oxygen utilization, hence the pO_2 gradient between the arterial and venous gas is decreased.
5. Elevated levels of carboxyhemoglobin.
6. Methemoglobinemia may be coexistent, depending on the source of gas exposure.
7. Chest X-ray—may be normal initially, later revealing signs of lung injury, respiratory distress syndrome (RDS), etc.
8. Pulmonary function tests—may show decreased forced vital capacity (FVC) and forced expiratory volume in 1 second (FEV1) levels.
9. CT brain or MRI—shows basal ganglia lesions, which are usually delayed findings.
10. ECG shows ischemia or infarction pattern.
11. Measurement of sulfide and thiosulfate levels may be useful in case of chronic low exposures.

Treatment

1. Immediate removal of the patient from the site of exposure, to a well-ventilated area with fresh air wash thoroughly with plenty of water or ask patient to have a shower immediately.
2. Administer high flow oxygen. Use of 100% oxygen inhalation is the mainstay of treatment of hydrogen sulfide poisoning. Use positive pressure ventilation in case of suspected acute lung injury.
3. Administer IV fluids, use normal saline or Ringer's lactate, which can combat hypotension.
4. In case of established hypotension, use vasopressors like dopamine as infusion.
5. Irrigation of the eyes to be done thoroughly to decrease evidence of eye irritation and possible ocular injury.
6. Based on ABG values, the acidosis needs to be corrected using sodium bicarbonate.

7. In case of evidence of bronchospasm, administer bronchodilators. Salbutamol acts on the beta-2 receptors to decrease the bronchospasm, which may be refractory to epinephrine administration.
8. In case of persistent brochospasm, use anticholinergics such as ipratropium bromide, which block the parasympathetic sites on bronchial smooth muscle with resultant brochodilation.
9. Consider racemic epinephrine aerosol for children, who develop stridor. Dose 0.25–0.75 mL of 2.25% racemic epinephrine solution in 2.5 cc water, repeat every 20 minutes as needed, cautioning for myocardial variability.
10. Inducing methemoglobinemia will help to combat the effects of H_2S toxicity. This is because the H_2S has more affinity to methemoglobin than to cytochrome oxidase and hence, the symptoms of toxicity can be reversed. Administer 0.2 mL/kg or 6 mg/kg of 3% sodium nitrite, (maximum 300 mg), IV over 2–4 minutes and obtain the methemoglobin levels 30 minutes later. If symptoms persist, the dose may be repeated. Monitor the patient for 24–48 hours after treatment.
11. In case of persistent neurologic findings, the patient may require hyperbaric oxygen therapy.

Watch out for side effects of sodium nitrite overdosage, which includes anxiety, cardiac dysrhythmias, circulatory failure, CNS depression, CV collapse, cyanosis, dyspnea, nausea, severe hypotension, tachycardia.

Complications

- Acute respiratory distress syndrome
- Acute myocardial infarction
- Delayed neuropsychiatric sequelae.

Prognosis

Long exposure to sublethal doses may result in long-term neurologic sequelae. However, short exposures even to high concentration, are not associated with any sequelae and the prognosis is good with adequate and early intervention.

SUGGESTED READING

Camphor Poisoning

1. Gibson DE, Moore GP, Pfaff JA. Camphor ingestion. Am J Emerg Med. 1989;7(1):41-43.
2. Kliegman RM, Behrman RE, Jenson HB, et al. Nelson Textbook of Pediatrics, 18th edition. Elsevier Health Sciences Division; 2007.
3. Khine H, Weiss D, Graber N, et al. A cluster of children with seizures caused by camphor poisoning. Pediatrics. 2009;123(5):1269-272.
4. Manoguerra AS, Erdman AR, Wax PR, et al. Camphor poisoning: An evidence—based practice guideline for out of hospital management. Clin Toxicol. 2006;44:357-70.
5. Siegel E, Wason S. Camphor toxicity. Pediatr Clin North Am. 1986;33(2):375-79.

Carbon Monoxide

1. Kliegman RM, Behrman RE, Jenson HB, et al. Nelson Textbook of Pediatrics, 18th edition. Elsevier Health Sciences Division; 2007.
2. Soghoian S. Pediatric carbon monoxide toxicity. www.medscape.com [Accessed June, 2012].

Hydrogen Sulfide

1. ATSDR. Medical management guidelines for hydrogen sulfide (H2S). www.cdc.gov.in
2. Human health effects of a toxic pollutant. Hydrogen sulfide. www.bredl.org [Accessed June, 2012].
3. Kliegman RM, Behrman RE, Jenson HB, et al. Nelson Textbook of Pediatrics, 18th edition. Elsevier Health Sciences Division; 2007.
4. Mandavia S. Hydrogen sulfide toxicity. www.medscape.com [Accessed June, 2012].
5. WHO 2003. Hydrogen sulfide human health aspects. Concise International Chemical Assessment Document 53.

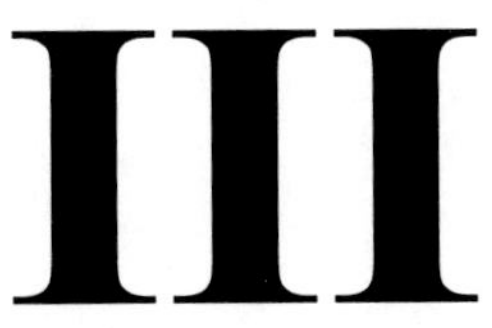

Section

Warfare

8 Chapter Biological Warfare

Biological warfare has been known from ancient times. However, these days, the methods have become more sophisticated and hard to diagnose and treat. Hence, it is very important to be aware, to prevent the spread and to protect oneself and the environment from these agents. These are also called 'weapons of opportunity', as they are rather easily available and can inflict a large number of casualties in a short span of time.

There are over 1,200 agents that can be used as biological weapons, by causing illness or death. However, only a few of them possess all the ideal characteristics, which are essential for an effective biological warfare agent. They should be easily procured, easy to carry; small amounts can cause maximum damage, should remain undetectable and can incapacitate thousands of people in a metropolitan area within a short period. They are colorless, odorless, undetectable and spread easily in the environment.

Germs of some various diseases like anthrax, plague, botulinum, tularemia, smallpox and viral hemorrhagic disease have been classified as category A biological warfare agents by the Center for Disease Control and Prevention (CDC), USA. Children are more susceptible to the effects of biological warfare, because of their higher respiratory rate, thinner skin and their developmental immaturity.

ROUTES OF SPREAD

1. By aerosol: Sprays used can easily disseminate in the environment and spread to cause the maximum damage by inhalation. The sprayed germs can enter the lungs and cause destruction, which can lead to instant death. It is the ideal weapon for mass destruction (WMD).

2. By water: The agents can be leaked into the city's drinking water systems after the treatment plant, so it enters the household and causes untold destruction.
3. By injection of the toxic agents: This cannot cause mass destruction, but can be used to create a scare in the community.
4. By use in explosive devices: The biological agents are usually destroyed by the explosion and barely 5% is left, hence is not an effective WMD.

DETECTION

Detection of biological agents are extremely difficult, because of their stealth characteristics. However, constant vigilance by the state is essential to get clues regarding the possibility of biological warfare attacks.

Doctors need to be aware of the symptoms and look out for early signs of suspicious disease symptoms following which the health authorities must be intimated immediately.

PROTECTION

Once suspected, it is very essential to protect oneself against the biological warfare agents. The use of personal protective equipments (PPEs) is essential to ensure non-exposure to the biological culprits.

1. Masks—wearing masks with high-efficiency particulate air (HEPA) filters, will protect against the inhaled toxic agents, by filtering out the germs. The masks need to be closely fitted to prevent any leaks on the face, which can nullify the protective effects.
2. Clothing—wearing clothes, which will fully cover the body parts is helpful, as the agents usually do not penetrate through the layers of clothing. Removal of clothing and washing off, the skin will be useful to eliminate at least 99.99% of the biological agents. However, certain exposed areas like hands and feet may still be exposed.
3. Protective clothing—masks, along with gowns, aprons, caps, gloves, eye pads and footwear can be used to completely cover all portions of the body. This is extremely cumbersome and can be recommended only for medical professionals treating the victims.

4. Immunization against known biological agents, like anthrax, tularemia, botulinum, plague, etc. may be useful for the military personnel who are at higher risk of exposure. Routine immunizations are not recommended for the general public.
5. Antibiotics may be administered orally or by intravenous (IV) route in suspected warfare patients even before the actual agent is identified.

Commonly used various agents are discussed, as it is essential to be aware and diagnose any unlikely signs and symptoms in the community.

ANTHRAX

Caused by the bacteria *Bacillus anthracis,* usually is an organism that affects the animals like horses, goats, sheep, cattle, etc. Humans get infected by contact with the infected animals, through skin inoculation. However inhalation of the spores, which are dormant in the soil or carcass can result in reactivation of the bacteria and is the most dangerous route for causing the highest casualties during attacks.

Cutaneous Anthrax

Cutaneous anthrax occurs when the spores enter via skin abrasions and cuts. The patient presents with fever, chills and headache. The site of inoculation turns into a tiny sore looking lesion, which progresses over the next 3–5 days to a fluid-filled blister. The organisms are teeming in this fluid. With appropriate treatment the vesicles heals with a blackened base, called 'eschar'. After about 2–3 weeks, the tissue separates, leaving behind a scar at the site.

Inhalation Anthrax

Inhalation anthrax occurs following the inhalation of the anthrax spores. Symptoms develop 1–6 days after exposure. The organisms get activated in the lungs. The patient presents with non-specific symptoms like fever, cough, malaise, headache, etc. A brief period of improvement may occur, but is followed rapidly by an accelerated phase with high fever, dyspnea, cyanosis and shock. About 50% have hemorrhagic meningitis. Chest X-rays may reveal widened mediastinum, mediastinal lymphadenopathy and pleural effusion. The Gram stain of the peripheral blood smear may show the anthrax organisms. Prompt and early aggressive treatment will reduce the mortality, which is usually around 95% within 2–3 days.

Inhalation anthrax does not spread from person to person. However, in case of terror attacks, the inhaled spores by individuals' from the aerosols can cause large-scale loss of life and casualty.

Gastrointestinal Anthrax

Gastrointestinal anthrax is a rare entity. This occurs when a person consumes infected, improperly cooked, meat. There is an incubation period of 1–3 days after which sores developed in the throat, difficulty in swallowing occurs associated with fever and neck swelling. Non-specific symptoms like fever, malaise and nausea may be associated with abdominal pain and diarrhea. Hemoptysis may also occur sometimes.

Investigations

A high-level of suspicion is essential, while treating these patients, especially when there is an outbreak of this type. In a mass casualty setting, always suspect agents of biological warfare.

1. Skin biopsy of the eschar reveals the presence of the anthrax bacteria.
2. Gram stain of the peripheral smear may show the bacteria during the accelerated stage of inhalation disease.
3. Chest X-ray—evidence of mediastinal enlargement, lymphadenopathy, pleural effusion.
4. Blood culture—organisms may be grown rapidly, within 6–24 hours, if suspected and the laboratory staff warned of the likelihood of anthrax.
5. Rapid diagnostic tests—enzyme-linked immunosorbent assay (ELISA), polymerase chain reaction (PCR) and direct fluorescent antibody (DFA) testing of the blood sample may aid in the early diagnosis. These tests are not available easily.

Treatment

1. Standard isolation practices to be employed for these patients.
2. Antibiotics are the mainstay of treatment.

3. Ciprofloxacin 10–15 mg/kg every 12th hourly given either orally or IV depending on the patient's condition and stability.
4. In case of intolerance to ciprofloxacin, the patient can be administered the combination treatment with doxycycline 2.2 mg/kg IV every 12th hourly plus clindamycin 10–15 mg/kg IV every 8th hourly plus penicillin G 400–600 K units/kg/day IV divided into 4th hourly doses.
5. Treatment is continued for at least 14 days or until the patient is stable, then continued on single drug orally, either ciprofloxacin or doxycycline for the completion of the course of 60 days.
6. Prophylaxis can be administered to at patients risk, using either ciprofloxacin or doxycycline orally for 60 days.
7. Immunization against anthrax is available, but is not done routinely. It is reserved for the military forces, who are likely to be exposed repeatedly. The dosing consists of 6 injections given over a period of 18 months, followed by annual booster shots.

PLAGUE

Plague is a bacterial infection caused by *Yersinia pestis* and can attack humans as well as animals. The bacterium is a facultative intracellular, gram-negative bacillus with a bipolar staining. Plague has been the scourge of mankind, having caused several pandemics over the centuries. The flea is the 'vector of spread' of the bacteria. When the flea bites the infected animal or the human being, the organism multiplies in the blood. The organism survives in the macrophages and hence is capable of travelling to distant sites in the body. When the infected flea attempts to bite again, it vomits clotted blood and bacteria into the bloodstream of the victim, which thus spreads the disease to other animals or humans. This is how the classical bubonic plague and the septicemic plague is spread. What is considered as a weapon for biological warfare is the pneumonic plague, which is the advanced stage during transmission. The organisms are inhaled and spread directly into the lungs and cause severe illness or death unless treated early. The aerosolized bacteria can be sprayed and contaminate the air, resulting in massive casualty and widespread loss of life.

Bubonic Plague

The symptoms are non-specific and the sudden onset of fever, malaise, cough and headache, may be associated with nausea. The lymph nodes enlarge and are painful within 1–8 days of infection. This is the earliest phase and as few as 1–10 organisms are adequate to cause the infection. If untreated, the organisms spread via lymphatics to the spleen, liver, lungs and even to the brain resulting in the next stage of the disease, i.e. the septicemic stage.

Septicemic Plague

Septicemic stage may be secondary to the bubonic plague or may occur as such after infection and the blood spread of the organisms. There is high fever with chills and shivering, nausea, vomiting and diarrhea. Skin tissues may be devitalized and skin bleedings may occur.

Pneumonic Plague

The organisms enter the lungs by inhalation or by seeding from the blood. The patient presents with cough and sometimes productive with blood-tinged sputum. Disseminated intravascular coagulation (DIC) and overwhelming sepsis can occur with a fulminant progression. Chest X-ray shows patchy consolidation. Patient can progress downhill rapidly unless aggressive treatment is started. This is the most serious form for biological warfare and large populations can be affected by spraying the organisms in the air.

Investigations

1. Lymph node aspiration and study would show the bipolar *Yersinia* organisms under the microscope.
2. In case of productive cough, the sputum may also show the presence of the bipolar organisms.
3. Culture of the sputum, blood or lymph node materials on a MacConkey TRA agar, may give results within 48 hours.
4. Chest X-ray may show patchy pneumonitis in case the respiratory symptoms predominate.

Treatment

1. Isolation of the patient with care against droplet spread. Patient to be isolated for 48–72 hours after start of treatment.

2. For the acute cases, especially the pneumonic plague, use of gentamicin 2.5 mg/kg IV every 8th hourly. Alternatively, use doxycycline 2.2 mg/kg IV every 12th hourly or ciprofloxacin 15 mg/kg every 12th hourly IV.
3. As prophylaxis, in susceptible contacts, use doxycycline 2.2 mg/kg every 12th hourly orally or ciprofloxacin 20 mg/kg every 12th hourly orally.
4. With adequate treatment, the buboes start decreasing in size after 10–14 days and can resolve without drainage.
5. Pneumonic plague needs aggressive antibiotic therapy within 18 hours of symptoms, else it is 100% fatal.
6. Bubonic plague is 60% fatal without treatment, while septicemic plague is 100% fatal without aggressive, early treatment.

TULAREMIA

Tularemia, a disease caused by a bacterium *Francisella tularensis,* can infect humans as well as animals. The organism has a high capacity to survive in the environment, hence it is a potential agent for biological warfare.

Francisella tularensis is highly infective. As less as 10 organisms are adequate to produce infection, which can be easily disseminated by aerosol spray. The symptoms are non-specific with fever, cough, headache and malaise.

In the ulceroglandular variety, the patient develops a sore, which is wide, usually up to an inch in size on the exposed part of the body. This is the classical feature of the disease and could be associated with chest pain, fever, abdominal pain, back pain or neck stiffness. Lymph node enlargement may occur singly or in groups and may be confused for buboes.

In the pneumonic type of tularemia, the organisms are inhaled from the aerosol spray. The lungs are infected, patient develops cough, which may be productive or non-productive associated with chest pain and symptoms mimicking pneumonia, has a fulminant course.

Investigations

1. Samples taken from the ulcer, blood or sputum can be cultured to grow the *F. tularensis* organism. However, it

needs to be grown on standard media that is enhanced with cysteine, for better isolation.

2. Rapid diagnostic methods like PCR, ELISA or serum agglutination assays may be used for early diagnosis.

Treatment

Standard isolation practices: Early aggressive treatment is essential especially in the pneumonic variety. Treatment is similar to that of plague as follows:

1. Administer for the acute cases, especially the pneumonic plague, use of gentamicin 2.5 mg/kg IV every 8th hourly. Alternatively, use doxycycline 2.2 mg/kg IV every 12th hourly or ciprofloxacin 15 mg/kg every 12th hourly IV.
2. As prophylaxis, in susceptible contacts, use doxycycline 2.2 mg/kg every 12th hourly orally or ciprofloxacin 20 mg/kg every 12th hourly orally.

Treatment needs to be continued for 14 days to ensure that no relapse occurs.

Prevention

Tetracycline or doxycycline used immediately after exposure within 24 hours, will be effective in case of inhaled toxins.

A vaccine against tularemia has been underdevelopment and has been shown to decrease the incidence of typhoidal and ulceroglandular types of disease.

SMALLPOX

Smallpox caused by organisms belonging to the variola virus species. It has an incubation period of 1–7 days after exposure therefore, resulting in large number of asymptomatic persons, who can spread the virus causing an epidemic outbreak of the dreaded disease.

The virus replicates in the respiratory system during the incubation stage and hence can be easily transmitted from person to person. During the primary viremia stage, the organisms get seeded in the liver and spleen, followed by the secondary viremia stage, when the organisms lodge and multiply in the skin, resulting in the classical exanthematous illness.

The infected person presents with fever, rigors, headache, vomiting and backache, associated with severe generalized malaise. Within 1–2 days, the macules appear on the face and back and progress in a centrifugal distribution, which distinguishes it from chickenpox. The macules progress to papules and to the pustules, from which they form scabs that may leave deep scars, which can result in permanent disfiguration of the victim. Mortality rate is around 30%, most of the causes is due to visceral involvement.

Investigations

A high index of suspicion is essential to diagnose this suspected agent of biological warfare. The clinical symptoms and examination will aid the diagnosis. Alongside, the fluid or tissue from the scabs can be collected and subjected to electron microscopy or culture, to visualize the organisms. Extra care should be exercised, while handling the materials from the scabs and papules.

Treatment

Supportive care is all that is required for treatment. The vaccine if administered early after exposure, may help in decreasing the incidence of smallpox following any external threat.

VIRAL HEMORRHAGIC FEVERS

Viral hemorrhagic fevers are a group of viruses belonging to the arbovirus groups. Viral hemorrhagic fevers are caused by four families of viruses as given below:

1. Arenaviridae (Lassa, Argentine, Bolivian, Brazilian, Venezuelan hemorrhagic fevers).
2. Bunyaviridae (Rift Valley, Crimean-Congo, Hantaan).
3. Filoviridae (Marburg, Ebola).
4. Flaviviridae (Yellow, Dengue, Kyasanur Forest, Omsk HFs).

The best known of the viral hemorrhagic fevers is Ebola virus. All the viruses have an incubation period ranging from approximately 3–8 days, with longer incubation only for certain types of viruses. The onset is usually acute with fever, headache, malaise and myalgia. This is usually followed by the appearance of hemorrhagic enanthems especially on the soft palate and petechial rash on the trunk and abdomen. This may be followed by epistaxis or frank hemoptysis, GI bleeds, hematemesis, melena, etc.

Respiratory distress may occur due to airway obstruction, pleural effusion or congestive heart failure. In severe cases, tremors, seizures and altered sensorium can occur. DIC and thrombocytopenia can be fatal complications.

Investigations

A high index of suspicion is essential. In case of clusters of cases, the likelihood of biological warfare must be suspected.

Most of the viruses of this group can be identified by culture of tissue from throat swabs, blood and sometime urine samples. Electron microscopy will help to detect the virus types. Serologic testing showing the 4-fold increase in the antibody titers will aid the diagnosis. Reverse transcriptase RNA polymerase detection can point to the diagnosis.

Treatment

Treatment is usually supportive and symptomatic.

1. Reversal or prevention of dehydration, hemoconcentration and renal failure.
2. Transfusion of platelets or fresh frozen plasma may be essential in case of DIC or severe hemorrhage.
3. Ribavirin may be useful especially in Lassa fever and certain other hemorrhagic fevers.

SUGGESTED READING

1. Dire DJ. Biological Warfare. www.medscape.com [Accessed June, 2012].
2. Kleigman RM, Behrman RE, Jenson HB, et al. Nelson Textbook of Pediatrics, 18th edition. Elsevier Health Sciences Division; 2007.

9 Chapter
Chemical Warfare

In today's world, the chances of chemical warfare are extremely high and children are usually easy and susceptible targets of these attacks. Hence, it is essential for all those who treat children to know how to recognize and deal with these situations. If treated early and adequately, the effects of these 'weapons of mass destruction' can be effectively negated. Children are more likely to be adversely affected due to the following reasons:

1. Thinner skin favoring easier and faster absorption.
2. Larger surface area of exposed skin per unit volume.
3. Lower volume of blood, hence small losses by vomiting, etc. translates to huge losses.

CATEGORIES OF WEAPONS OF MASS DESTRUCTION

The weapons of mass destruction (WMD) categories are as follows:

1. Nerve agents, e.g. sarin, soman, cyclosarin, tabun, VX.
2. Respiratory agents, e.g. chlorine, phosgene, diphosgene.
3. Cyanides.
4. Vesicating or blistering agents, e.g. mustard, lewisite.
5. Opioid agents.
6. Antimuscarinic compounds.
7. Vomiting agents, e.g. adamsite.
8. Riot control agents, e.g. pepper gas, cyanide.

Very rapid onset of symptoms is seen with the nerve agents and the respiratory agents, which are also called 'choking' agents.

The chemical agents are usually stored and transported as liquids and are utilized in liquid or aerosol form, for easy and rapid dispersion. The volatility of the agents is directly related to the temperature at which it is released, as at higher temperature, volatility is greater. The persistence of the liquid to remain in the liquid state is again related to the ambient temperature. The volatile liquids have a dual mode of action, via the dermal surface as well as via inhalation and are affected by the wind directions and enclosed spaces, both of which aggravate the effects of the agent. The persistent liquids are more absorbed via the skin. The amount of exposure to the agent and the area in which the liquid is deployed affect the extent to which the damage is caused.

Under temperate conditions, all nerve agents exist as volatile liquids, the highest volatility being noted in sarin and the least by VX. In comparable terms, the two agents are the ends of the spectrum like water and motor oil, indicating that VX has greater lipophilic properties and hence is extensively absorbed via the skin in comparison with sarin and is 100–150 times more toxic than sarin.

Pathophysiology

All the nerve agents are structurally similar to organophosphate pesticides malathion, hence their mechanism of action is similar to organophosphate compounds. The enzyme acetylcholinesterase is inhibited due to its phosphorylation by the nerve agents, with resultant paralyzing action of the cholinergic neurotransmitters in the body. They also directly bind the muscarinic and nicotinic receptors, antagonize the GABA neurotransmitters, while at the same time stimulating the N-methyl-D-aspartate (NMDA) receptors in the body. This is the important action, which produce the seizures and other pathologic features associated with the nerve gas inhalation.

Clinical Features

The symptoms and signs depend on various factors:

1. Dose of exposure.
2. Route of exposure.
3. Agent of exposure.

Inhalation of vapors results in toxic features almost immediately, within seconds. Even small doses are adequate to cause irritation, which may be local or systemic. At low doses, there occurs:

1. Ocular symptoms are blurred vision, watery eyes, eye pain, photophobia, meiosis nasal rhinorrhea.
2. Pulmonary symptoms are dyspnea, tightness in the chest, bronchoconstriction and bronchorrhea.

At high doses, vapor inhalation could result in the following:

1. Severe bronchoconstriction.
2. Fasciculations.
3. Hypersecretions from mouth and lungs.
4. Convulsions.
5. Respiratory arrest.

Minimal dermal exposure could result in the following:

1. Increased sweating, muscle fasciculations.
2. Nausea, vomiting, diarrhea, generalized weakness.

Severe dermal exposure could be rapidly fatal such as follows:

1. Loss of consciousness.
2. Convulsions.
3. Generalized fasciculations.
4. Flaccid paralysis.
5. Bronchoconstriction.
6. Death.

Exposure to liquid agents produces results as early as 30 minutes and may last up to almost 18–20 hours. The agents rapidly and completely penetrate through the dermal layers to produce various symptoms.

Mechanism of Action

Respiratory Tract

Muscarinic effects on the respiratory secretions, with profuse watery discharge and hypersecretions of the airways. Intense bronchoconstriction associated with stridor due to laryngeal muscle paralysis can interfere with respiratory functions. However, the nerve agents have a direct depressive action on the respiratory center and can be the main cause of early death. The smaller airway diameter, anatomic subglottic narrowing, relatively larger tongue size, less rigid ribs and trachea, make the child more vulnerable to the respiratory symptoms of toxicity. Also, the nerve agents cross the blood-brain barrier rapidly and children under 4 years of age, especially those with status epilepticus are at increased likelihood of death.

Cardiovascular System

Cardiovascular system actions depend on the balance between the nicotinic and muscarinic effects at the parasympathetic postganglionic cardiac nerve fibers. Tachycardia or bradycardia associated with arrhythymias, hyper or hypotension with or without atrioventricular (AV) blockade can occur. Prolonged QT interval with torsades de pointes have been noted. Superimposed hypoxia can cause tachycardia or tachydysrhythmias.

Ocular Signs

Ocular signs occur early due to the early penetration of the nerve gas into the conjunctiva with direct parasympathetic muscarinic effects. Constriction of the iris and ciliary muscle causes miosis, blurred vision, headache, pain nausea and vomiting. Epiphora due to lachrymal stimulation and redness of the eyes can also occur.

Musculoskeletal System

Musculoskeletal system is affected due to the paralyses of the neurotransmission at the neuromuscular junction, with resultant difficulty in walking, vague limb weakness, which can progress to fasciculations, followed by flaccid paralysis and apnea.

Neurological Symptoms

The neurological symptoms occur due to the cholinergic receptors being affected throughout the central nervous system (CNS). Headache, vertigo, paresthesia, insomnia, emotional depression followed by decreasing level of consciousness and generalized seizures may occur.

Investigations

1. Red blood cell (RBC) cholinesterase activity helps in the detection of suspected nerve gas toxicity. It is not totally reliable always. Reduction of 20%–25% below the reference levels may be associated with severe toxicity.

2. Plasma cholinesterase levels may have a better correlation with nerve gas exposure. However, as this is also produced by the liver, its levels may be reduced in liver disease or with infections. Hence, the plasma cholinesterase does not accurately predict severity of toxicity.

Under these conditions, decision to treat must be based on the clinical symptoms and findings together with the relevant history.

Treatment

In all cases of suspected chemical weapon agent exposure, whether in liquid or vapor form, it is essential for the emergency staff, the first responders to protect themselves by using personal protective equipments (PPE). The vapor contamination of the first responders does not continue beyond the 'hot zone' (area of exposure), while the liquid toxins remain deadly even beyond the hot zones. Hence, the hospital staff also need to be alerted to use PPEs, while handling these patients.

1. Decontamination of the patient, especially those exposed to liquid toxins. The 'triple decontamination' method is recommended. Thoroughly irrigate the exposed areas with water, followed by soap and water or 0.5% hypochlorite solution, to be followed by further rinsing with plenty of water for 5–10 minutes. No need to flush the eyes after vapor exposure.
2. In case of vapor toxicity, remove the clothes and jewelery after removal of patient from the hot zone.
3. Supportive care of the exposed patient, maintain the airway, provide oxygen and insert the intravenous (IV) cannula to maintain the circulation.
4. In case of altered sensorium, intubate and ventilate the patient. In case of muscarinic side effects of the nerve gas, the intubation may be difficult due to the excessive secretions. In these patients, first administer atropine before intubating and proceeding with other measure.
5. Specific treatment includes administration of Inj. atropine, which helps to dry the secretions and reduce the airway resistance, while at the same time decreases nausea, vomiting, abdominal cramps and bradycardia caused by

the muscarinic effects of the nerve gas. The doses may need to be repeated depending on the response, persistence of secretions or difficulty in intubation. Dose of atropine in children is 0.2 mg/kg either IV, intramuscular (IM) or endotracheal (ET). In case of severe symptoms, administer 0.5 mg/kg either IV/IM/ET.

Repeat atropine doses every 5–10 minutes, until dyspnea, secretions and resistance to ventilation have decreased and breathing is comfortable.

Do not use atropine IV in a hypoxic patient, as it may trigger ventricular fibrillation. In these situations, use the IM route for the initial doses.

6. To reverse the nicotinic effects, it is essential to administer pralidoxime, which belongs to the group of oximes. They bind to the phosphate moiety of the acetylcholinesterase, resulting in the release of the acetylcholinesterase (AChE) enzyme, which is reactivated thus. This drug has to be administered early during treatment, so that the maximal amount of AChE can be reactivated before it becomes totally inactive or dealkylated. Pralidoxime (P2AM) has the maximal effect on the neuromuscular junction. It has to be administered slowly to prevent untoward side effects like nausea, vomiting, blurred vision or hypertension. Dose in children will be 15–25 mg/kg IV over 30 minutes.

   Pralidoxime may need to be repeated in case of persistent symptoms or worsening of the symptoms, in which case it may be repeated every hourly for a total of three doses. IV infusions can be used for the second and third doses. In case the hypertension is aggravated due to P2AM, administer phentolamine 1 mg IV for children.

7. In case of persistent seizure activity despite giving atropine, administer a barbiturate, diazepam, lorazepam or even midazolam, to effectively abort the seizure activity, diffuse muscle twitching or if over one organ is involved.
8. In case of no response to medical treatment, it may be essential to provide hemodialysis for the unresponsive patient.

Guide to Discharge from Hospital

1. All nerve gas liquid exposure patients need to be monitored for at least 18 hours. If symptomatic, admit and monitor for at least 1 day.
2. Nerve gas vapor inhalants need to be monitored for at least 1 hour. As the peak effects would have been over most of the time before the patient has arrived at hospital, it may not be essential to further monitor after admission, unless the patient is symptomatic. No further worsening of the symptoms is usually expected and complete recovery is usually expected, as delayed neuropathy does not occur.

VESICATING OR BLISTERING AGENTS

Nitrogen mustard is an pungent-smelling liquid, which is highly soluble in oils, fats and organic solvents. It has the smell of garlic, onion or mustard. Nitrogen mustard has been used primarily as a chemotherapeutic agent, but it also has been used as a chemical weapon, since the World War I. It acts rapidly with predominantly dermatologic symptoms, hence has been considered a sudden onset WMD. At low ambient temperatures, it remains as a liquid, but when heated it vaporizes and gives out toxic fumes, which can be quite lethal.

Pathophysiology

The mustard agents produce their effects by various routes. They rapidly penetrate the dermal cells and generate an intermediate called episulfonium, which is highly toxic. This ion alkylates the deoxyribonucleic acid (DNA), ribonucleic acid (RNA) and cell protein, causing the cell disruption and cell death. The action is more rapid and effective in the presence of fluid, hence the dermal and hematopoietic cells are the most susceptible to alkylation.

The mustard also depletes the glutathione present in the cells, with resultant lipid peroxidation, loss of calcium homeostasis, inactivation of sulfhydryl-containing enzymes, all of which ultimately result in cell breakdown and death. Mustard vapor is highly toxic, probably more than cyanide gas. Mustard liquid in doses as little as 5 mL can cause serious toxicity. Symptoms and signs can occur anywhere from 1 to 24 hours after exposure, but usually can be noted by 4–6 hours.

Clinical Features

Due to its chemical properties, the mustard compounds are highly injurious and can cause irritation to the skin, eyes, respiratory tract, gastrointestinal tract (GIT) as well as the blood. High ambient temperature and humidity increase the effects of toxicity. While the vapors cause maximal damage to the respiratory tract, the liquids cause partial to full thickness dermal burns associated with blistering and vesicle formation. Moist areas like the axilla and groin are most susceptible to injury.

Dermal symptoms are commonly stinging and burning are usually followed by erythematous and edematous skin. The moist and thinner skin areas are likely to suffer more damage, with full thickness, deep bullae and ulcers that usually occur following exposure to higher concentrations. The lesions can be easily mistaken for those of scalded skin syndrome, but may be differentiated if clusters of cases occur simultaneously. The bulla fluid is sterile and non-contagious.

Ocular symptoms can be noted easily due to the extreme sensitivity of the eyes to the pungent vapor. Symptoms can be noted from 4 to 8 hours after exposure and usually present as burning or stinging sensation in the eyes, pain or blurred vision, photophobia, tearing and a foreign body sensation in the eyes. The signs point towards a local irritant, with eyelid edema, conjunctival congestion and edema, iritis, corneal abrasions, corneal ulcers and decreased visual acuity. Due to the likelihood of more severe exposure of the eyes to even milder levels of mustard exposure, the likelihood of ocular complications remains higher, with the possibility of corneal scarring and blindness occurring later.

Respiratory symptoms are the result of the direct irritant effect of the mustard vapors on the airways. The inflammation progresses downward, causing predominant symptoms referable to the upper respiratory tract, with the lower tract being rarely affected unless the exposure is severe and high levels of vapors are released. Hoarseness of voice may be a predominant symptom, associated with cough, sinus congestion or sinusitis, sore throat, etc. Occurrence of dyspnea and respiratory distress indicate lower airway compromise. Direct necrotic effect of the mustard can result in pseudomembrane formation followed by massive sloughing and obstruction. Delayed symptoms may also occur, even after several days after exposure.

Gastrointestinal symptoms are usually nausea, vomiting, diarrhea and weight loss, caused by the action of the mustard on the actively proliferating GI cells of the intestine.

Hematologic symptoms are unpredictable as the extent of bone marrow suppression cannot be accurately gauged or predicted. The bone marrow cells are destroyed and the early leukocytes and their precursors start getting destroyed 3–5 days after exposure. Anemia and thrombocytopenia occur, while the leukocytes are the lowest 2 weeks after exposure.

Investigations

No specific lab tests are available for diagnosis.

Treatment

Personal protective equipment must be used by all the emergency and medical caregivers of persons exposed to mustard agents.

1. Decontamination as soon as after exposure is the key to reducing the toxicity. It must be done within a few minutes after dermal exposure, as this prevents the mustard from causing irreversible damage to the dermal tissues.
2. Complete and thorough irrigation of the exposed areas with water, after removal of the contaminated clothing, followed by washing with 0.5% hypochlorite solution or soap and water, preferably alkaline soap, which helps to neutralize the mustard.
3. In cases with respiratory symptoms, the need for endotracheal intubation is high, as the membranes can slough and cause airway obstruction. Surgical airway may need to be created in case there is severe airway compromise, else insertion of the largest ET tube is recommended.
4. Monitor the fluid and electrolyte status and provide maintenance of fluids. Avoid overhydration.
5. In case of mustard-induced dermal burns, which are extremely painful, analgesics may need to be administered. In case of severe pain, narcotic analgesics may be administered.
6. In case of severe burns, tissue debridement, local topical antibiotics and antitetanus toxoid needs to be administered.
7. In case of ocular injury, rapid and thorough irrigation of the eyes, followed by antibiotic eye drops, corticosteroid eye

drops and mydriatics may be required. It is essential to seek the ophthalmologist's opinion at the earliest. Severe corneal injuries may take almost 2–3 months for complete healing to occur.

8. Symptoms beginning later than 12 hours after exposure usually do not progress in severity. These patients can be sent to home and asked to return in case of worsening of symptoms.

Guide to Discharge from Hospital

All patients, who are asymptomatic at admission need to be monitored for at least 12–18 hours after exposure. Those with severe dermal burns may need to be admitted and monitored in a burns unit, while those with severe respiratory symptoms will require ICU care. Most patients recover uneventfully, without residual damage. However, with severe exposure there may be some patients, who have residual ocular or respiratory symptoms that persist.

RESPIRATORY AGENTS

Respiratory agents act on the respiratory system and produce rapidly and usually severe reactions and toxic symptoms that could be rapidly fatal. This group of WMD's consist of gases, which are used in various industries and diffuse in the atmosphere rapidly.

Chlorine is a yellow green gas with a characteristic pungent acrid odor. It is easily soluble in water. Even at low levels, it causes irritation and can be distinguished rather easily. Phosgene is also a colorless gas with a pungent odor and is also used in industries. It is not easily soluble in water.

Pathophysiology

Chlorine gas is an airway irritant, as it is easily soluble in water and is denser than water. It is rapidly absorbed by the upper airway and causes early airway symptoms. The chlorine gas reacts with the fluid of the airway resulting in production of hydrochloric acid and free oxygen radicals, which cause tremendous irritation and symptoms in the airways.

Phosgene has a characteristic odor like that of newly mown hay. Upon inhalation, it reacts with the airway fluid and produces hydrochloric acid, which can cause some irritation in the upper airway. As this gas is not easily soluble in water, its actions are on the lower airways, which is secondary to acylation reactions on the pulmonary alveolar capillary membranes. It also causes an inflammatory reaction, which is secondary to the release of leukotrienes. The effects of phosgene inhalation are usually delayed due to which the victims tend to remain for longer duration in the hot zones.

Clinical Features

Chlorine gas exposure at levels as low as 1–10 ppm causes clinical symptoms of respiratory irritation. Stridor can be immediate, followed by wheezing, hemoptysis and later development of pulmonary edema. The respiratory symptoms are associated with tachycardia and hypertension, which is later followed by development of hypotension. The chlorine interferes with the metabolism causing metabolic acidosis, which may result from the cellular hypoxia. Ocular irritation with lachrymation, tearing or watering and a burning sensation may occur. At higher levels of gas exposure, there may be corneal burns and conjunctivitis. Liquid chlorine coming in skin contact can cause dermal burns and frostbite injury.

Phosgene causes slightly delayed symptoms, which are more related to the lower airway, symptoms may be delayed for up to 48 hours or may manifest within half an hour of exposure. Progressive pulmonary edema may cause severe dyspnea and secondary circulatory collapse. Right-sided heart failure may occur due to destruction of RBCs by the toxic fumes. Lactic acidosis will interfere with the cellular oxygen uptake. Dermal blisters, pain and inflammation can occur due to liquefied phosgene coming in contact with the skin. Ocular irritation, conjunctival burning and pain, conjunctivitis may occur. Phosgene inhalation causes exposure hemolysis with resultant plugging of the pulmonary capillaries and further aggravation of the pulmonary edema effects. It is directly hepatotoxic and also nephrotoxic with loss of functional nephrons. Inhalation of phosgene may result in nausea and vomiting.

Investigations

The diagnosis of chlorine or phosgene toxicity is usually a clinical diagnosis. Some of the following investigations may be helpful to guide the treatment:

1. Complete blood count (CBC), blood glucose levels and serum electrolytes—will guide the treatment and fluid administration guidelines.
2. Pulse oximetry—to monitor the oxygenation levels.
3. Arterial blood gas (ABG)—to monitor the pulmonary functions.
4. Acid-base imbalances may be noted in chlorine exposure. Hyperchloremic acidosis may be found.
5. Chest X-ray—evidence of pulmonary edema with patchy infiltrates and hilar enlargement are late findings.

Treatment

The treatment is only supportive. There is no specific antidote available for chlorine and phosgene toxicity as follows:

1. Decontamination of the victim must be performed at low ambient temperature. Wash the exposed areas thoroughly with running water for 2–3 minutes, followed by washing with soap and water and thorough rinsing again.
2. The contaminated clothes must be removed immediately and placed in double bags.
3. Irrigate the exposed eyes for atleast 15–20 minutes.
4. Evaluate the airways and provide support in the form of intubation in case of altered sensorium.
5. Maintain the oxygen supply and establish the IV access to provide the fluids.
6. In case of stridor following exposure, administer racemic epinephrine: 0.25–0.75 mL of 2.2% racemic epinephrine in 2.5 mL water. It can be repeated every 20 minutes depending on the patient response, along with cardiac monitoring.
7. In case of bronchospasm, aerosol medications and bronchodilators are recommended for faster response.
8. In case of phosgene exposure, steroids are indicated to decrease the intense inflammation and pulmonary edema

that may occur. Other drugs that may be used in case of pulmonary involvement are terbutaline, N-acetylcysteine, aminophylline, etc.

9. Prophylactic antibiotics are not indicated, unless there is evidence of occurrence of pneumonia following exposure.
10. No role for diuretics in the treatment of pulmonary edema.
11. In case of frostbite lesions, place the exposed skin in warm water or gently wrap the part in blankets, while encouraging the exercise and movement of the affected parts.
12. In case of dermal burns, they should be treated as thermal burns, with extra caution as the children are more susceptible to toxicity due to the larger body surface area.
13. In case of ocular exposure, after thorough irrigation, the eyes must be checked for corneal ulcers and treated accordingly.

Guide to Discharge from Hospital

1. Victims of chlorine exposure, if asymptomatic can be discharged after checking and follow-up and should be asked to report immediately in case of any new symptoms developing.
2. In case of ocular exposure to chlorine, the patient must be revaluated after 24 hours.
3. In case of severe respiratory symptoms, the patient has to be admitted and treated until the symptoms subside.
4. Long-term follow-up for respiratory symptoms is indicated to rule out chlorine-induced reactive airways dysfunction syndrome (RADS), which can persist up to 12 years.
5. Following phosgene exposure, the patient must be treated symptomatically and must be reviewed after 24 hours, as delayed symptoms are known to occur. Patients with mild symptoms may be discharged after reassessment.

CYANIDE POISONING

Cyanide gas toxicity can be rapid and fatal. The inhaled vapors begin to act within few seconds to minutes after exposure, especially if it is in an enclosed space.

Cyanide in the liquid form is rapidly absorbed via the skin, producing its effects from few minutes to 1 hour later. Occasionally, especially in toddlers who display hand-to-mouth behavior, cyanide may be ingested.

Pathophysiology

Cyanide is a cellular poison, which is rapidly volatile and extremely deadly even in small quantities.

Cyanide gas is highly volatile, hence rapidly disperses. Its maximal effect will be felt only when inhaled in a closed environment. Cyanide gas inhibits the cellular enzyme cytochrome a3, thus interfering with mitochondrial oxidative metabolism with lactic acidosis formation. Decreased peripheral oxygen utilization results in cellular anoxia, elevated anion gap, metabolic acidosis and elevated mixed venous oxygen saturation value.

Clinical Features

Initially there are non-specific symptoms of excitement, dizziness, headache, nausea and vomiting, which can progress to lethargy, convulsions and loss of consciousness.

Bradycardia, cardiac arrhythmias, may follow the intial phase with tachycardia and transient hypertension. The bradycardia may be associated with hypotension, which may progress to death.

Shortness of breath associated with chest tightness and increased respiratory rate may be noted early after exposure. As the exposure increase, the respirations may become slow and gasping. Central cyanosis may not occur. Due to the anaerobic respiration, there is metabolic acidosis. Pulmonary edema may occur later.

Direct ocular contact with cyanide liquid will cause eye irritation, swelling and conjunctivitis. Systemic absorption via the skin is more at higher ambient temperatures and relative humidity. Children are more susceptible to dermal absorption due to the thinner skin and larger surface area to weight ratio.

Investigations

1. Complete blood count (CBC), blood glucose and electrolytes.
2. Anion gap to detect metabolic acidosis.
3. Pulse oximetry—to measure the oxygen saturation.
4. ECG in all leads—to note any cardiac dysrhythmias.

5. Venous blood gases—may show abnormally high levels of oxygen due to the inadequate tissue utilization of glucose.
6. Serum lactate and serum cyanide levels can be estimated.
7. Blood methemoglobin levels—should be less than 20%–30% in children.

Treatment

Provide immediate triage and maintain the airway, breathing and circulation of the victim. When symptomatic, provide the specific antidote, while decontaminating the victim. Provide 100% oxygen for inhalation.

1. Decontamination of the victim includes immediate removal from the hot zone, remove the contaminated clothes and bedding. Wash thoroughly the exposed parts with running water for 2–3 minutes, wash with soap and water, then rinse thoroughly. Examine the mouth, as children do tend to have hand-mouth behavior.
2. Care providers must be suitably protected, as the cyanide easily penetrates through the skin. It is essential to use butyl rubber gloves, which are also penetrated by the cyanide after sometime.
3. The specific antidote for cyanide poisoning is amyl nitrite. Break a pearl of this and place it under the victim's nose or near the Ambu valve intake and allow to inhale for 30 seconds. Use a fresh amyl nitrite pearl for every 3 minutes.
4. In a symptomatic patient, once the IV access has been established, stop the amyl nitrite inhalation and provide IV infusion of the drug.

   Dose: 0.12–0.33 mL/kg given as an infusion over at least 5 minutes. Monitor the blood pressure during infusion and watch for hypotension. Follow-up immediately with IV sodium thiosulfate at the rate of 1.65 mL/kg of a 25% solution. The IV sodium nitrite acts to remove the cyanide from the cells, which subsequently binds with the hemoglobin to form methemoglobin.
5. If the methemoglobin levels are dangerously high (> 20%–30%) it can be reversed by administration of 1% methylene blue. This dissociates the cyanide from the hemoglobin and sends it back into the cells.

6. Continuous cardiac monitoring will detect the occurrence of dysrhythmias. In case there is associated acidosis, administer sodium bicarbonate IV at the rate of 1 mg/kg.
7. In case of apnea, seizures shock, cardiac arrhythmia and pulmonary edema. The appropriate symptomatic treatment must be given.
8. In case of cyanide ingestion do not induce emesis. In case patient is alert, gastric lavage may be performed after administration of activated charcoal.
9. Any other injuries or complications should be treated accordingly.

Guide to Discharge

1. Asymptomatic patients can be discharged after 6 hours of observation.
2. For all symptomatic patients, they need to be admitted and treated with continuous monitoring. Discharge to be considered after all symptoms are stabilized.
3. Follow-up and evaluation of symptomatic patients for ischemic CNS and CVS damage. Late CNS complications include occurrence of Parkinsonian like symptoms.

SUGGESTED READING

1. Arnold JL. Chemical Warfare. www. medscape.com [Accessed July, 2012].
2. Childrens Medical Center, Washington DC. Patient care guidelines. www.dcchildrens.com [Accessed July, 2012].
3. Kleigman RM, Behrman RE, Jenson HB, et al. Nelson Textbook of Pediatrics, 18th edition. Elsevier Health sciences division; 2007.

IV

Section

Venoms

10 Chapter Snakebite

SNAKEBITE ENVENOMATION IN CHILDREN

Most snakebites are caused by non-poisonous varieties of snakes. There are over 3,000 species of snakes worldwide. Out of these only 15% are considered to be dangerous to human beings. India is home for 216 species of snakes, out of which the majority are non-poisonous.

Snakes can be classified into the following superfamilies:

1. Henophidia—includes the boas, pythons and related species.
2. Typhlopidae—these are the blind snakes.
3. Xenophidia—consists of several families as given below:
   i. Viperidae—which is the largest family of venomous snakes, found in various parts of Africa, America, Europe and Asia.
      a. Subfamily crotalidae, which includes pit vipers, rattlesnakes and copperheads, which inhabit the dry grassy areas and rocky hillsides.
   ii. Elapidae—is the next largest species of venomous snakes and includes the coral snakes, which have colored rings on the body. Their fangs are located in front of the mouth. The cobra and krait belong to this family. There are at least 200 species belonging to this family, out of which at least 20 species are dead.
   iii. Colubridae—all other varieties of snakes belong to this family. They have their fangs at the back of the mouth.
   iv. Hydrophiidae—includes the sea and water snakes.

Pathophysiology

The fangs or teeth of the snake are located on the upper jaw. The venom is produced and stored in paired glands below the eye and is discharged via the fangs, which are hollow. There are pits on the skin surface near the nostril, which respond to the heat emitted by the prey. Depending on the snake, the amount of venom varies. It also depends on the time elapsed, since the last bite and the degree of threat perceived by the snake. They inject the venom through the fangs. The purpose of injecting the venom is multifold:

1. It incapacitates the prey.
2. It aids the digestion of the tissues of the prey.
3. Acts as a deterrent to the predators.

The venom is usually watery and contains enzymes, which have destructive properties. These enzymes are mainly collagenase, protease, arginine ester hydrolase, hyaluronidase, phospholipase, etc. The enzyme concentration varies in different venoms and is responsible for the different patterns of tissue or organ damage that occurs (Fig. 10.1).

Mechanism of Action of the Venoms

The mechanism of action of the venoms is as follows:

- Cobra: neurotoxin
- Krait: combination of neurotoxin and hemolysin
- Viper: combination of hemorrhagin and hemolysin

Local Effects of Venoms

- Local edema, increased capillary leak of tissue fluid
- Coagulopathy
- Interstitial fluid leak in the lungs
- Myonecrosis and myoglobinuria
- Lactic acidosis
- Renal damage
- Cardiac failure.

Symptoms

It is essential to know, whether the snakebite was from a poisonous or a non-poisonous snake.

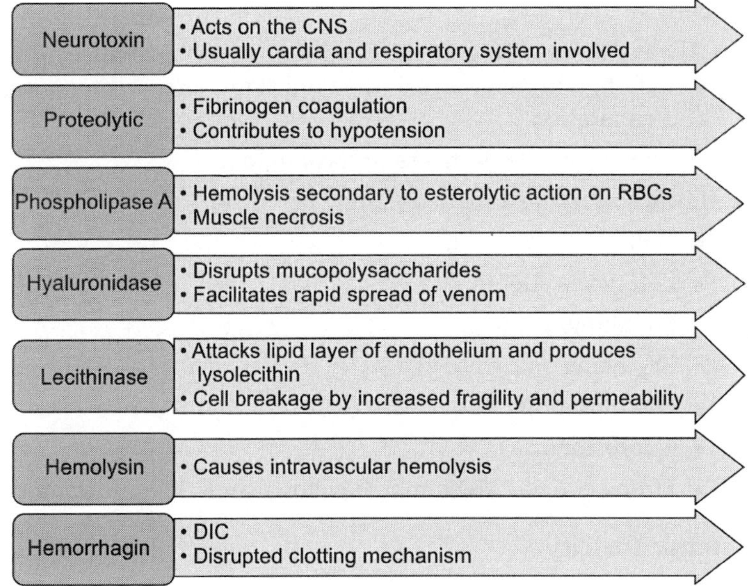

Fig. 10.1: Constituents of venom

In case of non-poisonous snakes, there are:

1. No distinct fang marks.
2. No local signs of swelling, edema pain or blistering.
3. No progressive symptoms noted. But this may not always be accurate. After biting, the snakes are usually present around the site, at least within 20 feet. Assess the time elapsed between biting and presentation at the medical facility.

Symptoms common to all snakebites:

1. Local swelling, edema, pain, paresthesia associated with systemic symptoms.
2. Fang marks may be seen at bite site.
3. Local tissue destruction, like streaking pitting, erythema or discoloration.
4. Evidence of bleeding, epistaxis, hemoptysis.
5. Generalized weakness.

Determine any history of drug allergy, drug consumption or any other allergies in the patient.

Signs

1. Always assess the general condition of the patient at presentation, with reference to the vital signs, airway, breathing and circulation.
   - Look for the fang marks or local injury.
2. Local soft tissue destruction may be noted:
   - Bullae
   - Soft tissue edema
   - Streaking
   - Erythema
   - Discoloration
   - Contusions
   - Pitting edema, which may develop over 6–12 hours later.

Systemic Toxicity

- Petechiae
- Epistaxis
- Hemoptysis
- Paresthesias and dysesthesias
- Hypotension.

Differentiation Based on Symptoms

Late onset envenomation has to watched for, as symptoms may develop from 6 to 12 hours after the bite has occurred. The difference between viperine and elapid envenomation is given in Table 10.1.

The extent of envenomation needs to be graded into:

1. Mild local pain, edema, no evidence of systemic toxicity and normal laboratory investigations.
2. Moderate to severe local pain, edema greater than 12 inches surrounding the wound along with systemic toxicity signs like nausea and vomiting plus abnormal platelet count and hematocrit.

Table 10.1: Difference between viperine and elapid envenomation

Viperine envenomation (vipers, rattlesnake, etc.)	Elapid envenomation (cobra, krait)
Swelling and local pain present	Swelling and local pain present
Local lymph nodes enlarged and tender due to presence of venom in lymphatics	Local necrosis and blistering especially with cobra
Epistaxis, bleeding gums and bleeding from other orifices	Descending paralysis starting from the cranial nerves, includes ptosis, diplopia—difficulty in focusing, heavy eyelids, smell and taste altered
Acute abdomen, suggestive of massive retroperitoneal hemorrhage	Numbness around lips, pooling of saliva, airway obstruction, bulbar paralysis, respiratory failure
Hypotension due to hypovolemia or vasodilatation	Hypoxia due to inadequate ventilation, cyanosis, altered sensorium and coma
Passing reddish urine, no urine output, backache suggestive of early renal failure or retroperitoneal bleed	Paradoxical respiration due to intercostal muscle weakness
Asymmetrical pupils, lateralizing neurological signs, may indicate intracranial bleeding	Pain abdomen, which may indicate submucosal bleeds in the stomach
Parotid swelling, subconjunctival hemorrhage, conjunctival edema may be associated with severe muscle pain due to rhabdomyolysis	Early morning paralysis, which can be mistaken for a stroke, is indicative of a krait bite

3. Severe generalized bleeding diathesis as seen by petechiae, ecchymoses, blood-tinged sputum plus systemic signs like hypotension, renal dysfunction, hypoperfusion along with abnormal prothrombin time, partial thromboplastin time, etc.

The grading should be a dynamic process as the patients' condition will change overtime, based on the treatment initiated, as well as depending on the effects of the venom.

Investigations

1. Twenty minutes whole blood clotting time (20WBCT)—is the most reliable bedside indicator of coagulation in the patient and is superior to the capillary tube method. This is the preferred method in snakebites.
    a. A few mL of fresh venous blood is kept in a new clean dry glass test tube vessel and left at ambient temperature for 20 minutes. After 20 minutes, gently tilt the tube; if the blood is still liquid, this indicates incoagulable blood.
    b. Repeat the test every 30 minutes from admission for 3 hours and then every hour after that; if the blood is still incoagulable, use the 6 hours cycle for deciding the need for repeat of antisnake venom (ASV) doses.

Other Tests

1. Hemoglobin (Hb), packed cell volume (PCV), peripheral smear—evidence of hemolysis.
2. Coagulation parameters—platelet count, prothrombin time (PT), activated partial thromboplastin time (APTT), fibrinogen degradation production (FDP), D-dimer.
3. Urine test—proteinuria, red blood cells (RBCs), hemoglobinuria, myoglobinuria.
4. Serum creatinine, urea, potassium.
5. Electrocardiography (ECG) in all 12 leads—to detect any electrolyte disturbances.
6. X-ray, ultrasound sonography (USG) abdomen—to detect any internal bleeds.
7. Computed tomography (CT) scan.

Treatment

First Aid Treatment

1. Treat the patient 'RIGHT'.
    a. 'R'—reassure the patient.
    b. 'I'—immobilize the affected part in a similar manner to a fractured limb.
    c. 'GH'—get to hospital immediately.

d. 'T'—tell the doctor about any systemic symptoms that may have manifested enroute to hospital.

2. Do not wash the wound. This stimulates the flow in the lymphatics and increase the flow of the venom.
3. Do not apply the tourniquet as this gives the patient a false sense of assurance. There is also an increased likelihood of limb ischemia and necrosis due to excessive pressure of the tourniquet. Procoagulant enzymes can cause distal clotting of blood and can result in embolism when the tourniquet is released.
4. Wherever possible, pressure immobilization by use of a crepe bandage, correctly applied will help to decrease the flow of the venom.

Assess the Patient on Arrival

1. ABC to be stabilized—maintain the airway, ensure adequate breathing and maintain the circulation by establishing the IV access.
2. If there is evidence of bite with the skin broken, give injection—tetanus toxoid.
3. Routine use of antibiotics is not recommended. Use if there is evidence of cellulitis or tissue necrosis.

Diagnosis Phase

1. Identify the snake where possible. Have the victim bring the snake to hospital, if it has been killed.
2. Keep all patients under observation for at least 24 hours.
3. Fang marks alone do not help in diagnosis. Some snakes grow reserve fangs in case the main ones break off.
4. Ask for any traditional medicine that has been used as it can cause misleading symptoms.
5. Ask the exact time of the bite as it can give an idea about progression of symptom.

Pain Management

The victims can suffer from excruciating pain following the snakebite (Table 10.2). This can be treated with administering pain killers that can be given orally. Paracetamol 10 mg/kg every 4–6 hours may be sufficient in milder cases. In more severe pain, it may be necessary to administer mild opiates like tramadol 50 mg orally or intravenously (IV).

In case the patient has come with a tourniquet, release the same gently after checking the distal pulse. Sudden removal of the tourniquet can cause a sudden massive release of venom resulting in neurological paralysis, respiratory distress, hypotension due to vasodilatation, etc. Hence, it is essential to have all resuscitation equipment close by before removal of the tourniquet. Alternatively, apply the blood pressure (BP) cuff and slowly deflate it.

Table 10.2: Simple guide to differentiate the effects of the venoms

Features	Cobra	Krait	Russel viper	Saw-scaled viper	Hump-nosed viper
Local pain/ tissue damage	Yes	No	Yes	Yes	Yes
Neurological signs/ptosis	Yes	Yes	Yes	No	No
Hemostatic abnormalities	No	No	Yes	Yes	Yes
Renal damage	No	No	Yes	No	Yes
Response to ASV	Yes	Yes	Yes	Yes	No
Response to neostigmine	Yes	No	No	No	No

General Thumb Rule

1. Hemostatic abnormalities indicate viper bites.
2. Cobras and kraits produce more of neurological manifestations.
3. Vipers can produce presynaptic neurological symptoms, hence the response to neostigmine is doubtful in these cases.

ANTISNAKE VENOM

Indications

Indications for use of antisnake venom (ASV):

- Shock
- Incoagulable blood
- Spontaneous systemic bleeding
- Acute renal failure
- Myoglobinuria
- Extensive progressive tissue swelling.

No test dose needs to be given before administration of ASV, as it has not been found to have any predictive value in detecting anaphylactoid or late serum reactions. In fact the test may presensitize the patient to ASV and cause greater risk, as the sensitization reactions are complement mediated and not immunoglobulin E (IgE) mediated.

Rationale: Administer adequate ASV to neutralize the average amount of injected venom, which could vary from 5 to 63 mg of venom.

1. Dose: initial dose is 8–10 vials of ASV for neurotoxic or hemostatic actions.
2. Each vial is 10 mL of reconstituted ASV, which has a neutralizing capacity of about 6 mg of venom.
3. It can be administered as a slow IV injection at 2 mL/min or as an infusion of ASV diluted in 5–10 mL/kg body weight of isotonic saline or glucose.
4. ASV to be administered over 1 hour, at a constant rate.
5. Patient needs to be closely monitored for at least 2 hours.
6. No infusion of ASV into the local area or site of bite.
7. ASV is available in two forms: liquid and lyophilized forms:
   a. Liquid ASV.
      - Cold chain and refrigeration needed
      - Shelf life is 2 years.

b. Lyophilized ASV.
    - Does not need cold chain maintenance
    - Available in powder form
    - Useful in rural areas with inconsistent power supply.

Other Indications for ASV

1. Evidence of systemic envenomation—20WBCT positive or spontaneous systemic or gingival bleeds; other lab parameters providing evidence of altered hemostatic mechanism.
2. Evidence of neurotoxicity—ptosis, muscle paralysis, external ophthalmoplegia, head drop, etc.
3. Cardiovascular (CVS) abnormalities—arrhythmias, hypotension, shock, abnormal ECG.
4. Persistent and severe vomiting or pain abdomen.
5. Severe local envenomation—local swelling, involving over half the limb or rapid extension of the swelling over a few hours.

Prophylaxis for Prevention of ASV Reactions

Antisnake venom can cause anaphylactic reactions, hence it may be a routine in some hospitals to administer it under cover of antihistamines. There are two possible regimes recommended, which need to be given before ASV injection.

1. 2 mg/kg of hydrocortisone plus 0.1–0.3 mg/kg of antihistamine [10 mg amp chlorpheniramine maleate IV/25 mg amp promethazine HCl intramuscular (IM)].
2. 0.25–0.3 mg adrenaline 1:1,000 solution given subcutaneously.

Special Situations

1. When the patient arrives late: Usually after several days, the patient may present to the hospital with acute renal failure. The need for ASV is determined by doing a 20WBCT, if there is evidence of coagulopathy, administer ASV, else no need to give ASV. Aggressively, treat the renal failure with dialysis and nephrologist consultation.
2. When the patient arrives late with neurotoxic symptoms like respiratory distress or ptosis, it is better to administer at least

8–10 vials of ASV to neutralize any unbound venom. Also vigorous respiratory support is essential.

Treatment of Anaphylaxis to ASV

1. Anaphylaxis can be life-threatening and can occur rapidly during ASV administration. It is essential to always have adrenaline easily available and administer it in case of any sign of adverse reactions.
2. Stop ASV immediately.
3. Administer 0.01 mg/kg of adrenaline IM.
4. For longer protection against adverse reactions, administer: hydrocortisone 2 mg/kg IV plus 0.2 mg/kg chlorpheniramine maleate IV (alternatively pheniramine maleate 0.5 mg/kg/day IV or promethazine HCl 0.3–0.5 mg/kg IM).
5. If the patient's condition has not improved after 10–15 minutes, administer a second dose of adrenaline 1:1,000 IM. This can be given as a third dose if necessary after 15–20 minutes. Usually two doses are adequate. IV fluids may need to be given rapidly if hypotension is associated.
6. Restart the ASV slowly for 10–15 minutes, while closely observing the patient. IV fluid rate to be adjusted accordingly.
7. Use of adrenaline is recommended early, as the IM route results in rapid elevation of the blood levels, within 8 minutes and gives the required responses rapidly.
8. Adrenaline given by the IV route is extremely rare, only in case of life-threatening reactions and with no response to IM adrenaline. It has to be given only with the support of ventilator procedure being easily available.
9. Late reactions can be covered by use of oral prednisone 0.7 mg/kg/day along with oral antihistamines.

Neurotoxic Envenomation

Neostigmine is useful in cases of postsynaptic neurotoxins like those of the cobra. It is an anticholinesterase, which increases the life of acetylcholine and therefore, causes reversal of respiratory symptoms and neurotoxic symptoms. However, its use in presynaptic neurotoxins is limited.

To determine the usefulness in cases of neurotoxin envenomation, use the neostigmine test. Administer 0.04 mg/kg of neostigmine IM along with injection atropine 0.05 mg/kg IV. Closely observe the patient for 1 hour to detect the effect of neostigmine. Neostigmine administration is followed by visible improvement, if any within 30 minutes after administration.

Watch the following to note any improvement:

1. Single breath count.
2. Diameter of iris uncovered by the eyelids.
3. Interincisor distance, between the upper and lower incisors.
4. Length of time the upward gaze can be maintained.
5. Pulmonary function tests: Forced expiratory volume in 1 second (FEV1) or forced vital capacity (FVC), if available.

If improvement in any of the neurological signs is noted, continue to administer the neostigmine along with atropine IV over the next 8 hours by infusion. If no improvement is noted after 1 hour, the neostigmine should be stopped.

Recovery Stage

If adequate antivenom has been administered, the patient will show evidence of recovery.

- Spontaneous bleeding stops by 15–20 minutes
- Postsynaptic neuronal signs improve in 30 minutes
- Shock improves by 30 minutes
- Blood coagulability restored in 6 hours
- Active hemolysis and rhabdomyolysis—improves in few hours
- Urine color normal within few hours
- Presynaptic neurotoxic symptoms improve within few hours.

Repeat Doses of ASV for Neurotoxic Envenomation

In case, the initial loading dose of ASV has not brought about the desired results in symptom reduction or the patient has worsened symptoms or has gone into respiratory failure, then it is essential to administer the repeat dose of ASV. This should be the same as the initial amount of ASV administered, i.e. 10 vials. This is the maximum dose that can be given for neurotoxic envenomation.

In case the patient has developed respiratory failure and is intubated and on the ventilator, there is no further need for ASV, as recovery thereafter would only depend on the body production.

Hemostatic Envenomation

Antisnake venom administration every 6 hours, as the liver is unable to generate the coagulation factors in less than 6 hours. Loading dose of ASV is administered over 1 hour.

Wait for 6 hours before repeating the coagulation tests. In case of persistent disturbance, administer the next dose of ASV over 1 hour, thus continue the cycle of ASV and coagulation parameters, until it is restored to normal. The repeat doses are half the original doses, i.e. 5–10 vials need to be given.

Once the coagulation profile has become normalized, there is no further need to administer ASV. There is no role of prophylactic ASV administration to prevent the recurrence of clotting abnormality. If there is persistence of the clotting abnormality despite recurrent doses of ASV, which have numbered over 30 vials, it is essential to relook at the cause of the coagulopathy. In these circumstances, it may be essential to administer fresh frozen plasma (FFP).

Hypotension After Snakebite

The pathophysiology of the hypotension is multifactorial—volume loss due to hemorrhage, vasodilatory effect of the venom or due to the direct cardiotoxic effect of the venom on the heart. It can be detected by recoding the blood pressure in the supine and the erect posture and noting a drop on change in posture.

These patients need to be administered plasma expanders and in case of generalized capillary permeability, there is need for vasoconstrictors like dopamine 5–10 μg/kg/min.

Surgical Intervention

Surgical debridement of the necrotic tissue is indicated to improve healing. However, the role of fasciotomy is seldom indicated as the intracompartmental pressure adequate to cause capillary collapse seldom occurs. There is no role of surgery to reduce or remove the venom.

Persistent or Severe Bleeding

Usually, the administration of sufficient amounts of ASV will reduce the bleeding. However, sometimes, the bleeding continues and will need further treatment. In these situations, it may be essential to administer FFP, cryoprecipitate or whole blood. However, it is essential to normalize the coagulation before administration of FFP, whole blood or any other coagulation factors.

Renal Failure

Renal failure is a frequent complication of Russell's viper and hump-nosed pit viper bites, mainly due to direct nephrotoxicity, intravascular hemolysis, disseminated intravascular coagulation (DIC), rhabdomyolysis and hypotension.

Suspect renal failure in the following situations:

- Oliguria
- Anuria
- Serum creatinine is more than 5 mg/dL or rising by more than 1 mg/day
- Blood urea more than 200 mg/dL
- Serum potassium more than 5.6 mmol/L
- Metabolic acidosis
- Clinical signs of uremia.

Treatment

1. Renal function deterioration needs to be treated aggressively.
2. Peritoneal dialysis can be initiated at the earliest indication of renal failure.
3. In case of hyperkalemia or hypotension, hemodialysis may be preferred.
4. Refer the patient to a nephrologist for further management.

Prognosis

- Depends on several factors
- 5A's that can predict the outcome (Fig. 10.2)
- In case of early aggressive therapy, full recovery is the rule

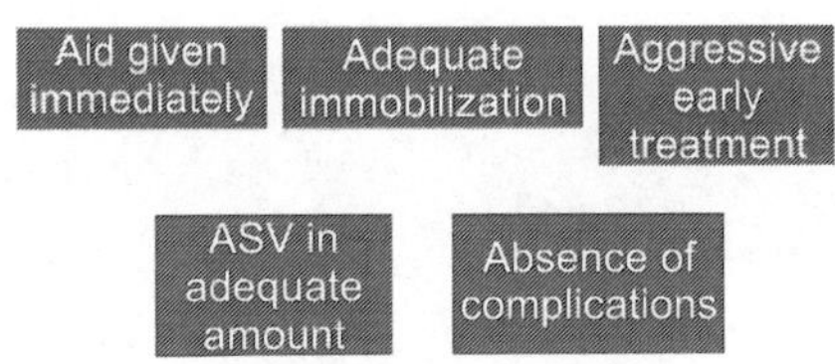

Fig. 10.2: Predictors of outcome

- Local complications of the envenomation may occur
- Death occurs in less than 1:5,000 cases, but varies depending on the factors enumerated above.

SUGGESTED READING

1. Adhisivam B, Mahadevans. Snakebite envenomation in India: A rural medical emergency. Indian Pediatrics. 2006;43:553-54.
2. Indian National Snakebite Protocol. Designed by the Indian National Snakebite Consultation Meeting, 2nd August 2007.
3. Kleigman RM, Behrman RE, Jenson HB, et al. Nelson Textbook of Pediatrics, 18th edition. Elsevier Health sciences division; 2007.
4. South Asian Cochrane Network and Center, Toxicology Special Interest Group, Dept of Medicine, 2012. Interventions for snakebites: An overview.

11 Chapter — Scorpion Stings

SCORPION STING ENVENOMATION

Scorpion stings are common in India, especially during the hot summer months, when they tend to move out to cooler areas. They get transported to distant areas by accidentally crawling into baggage, shoes or other containers and reach places, which are distant from their original habitat.

There are approximately 1,500 species of scorpions worldwide out of which about 50 pairs are dangerous to humans. They have a flattened body due to which it is easy to hide in cracks and small crevices. The color varies from brown to black and makes for convenient camouflage. They vary in size from 1 to 20 cm in length.

There are different families of scorpions, which are found in different parts of the world and have varied characteristics.

Classification

A. Family Buthidae—characteristic feature of this is the triangular-shaped sternum, thin body, weak looking pincers and thick tail. The majority of the lethal scorpions belong to this family.

This family consists of eight genera:

1. *Buthus*—which is found in the Mediterranean are ranging from Spain to the Middle East.
2. *Parabuthus*—abundant in Western and Southern Africa.
3. *Mesobuthus*—commonly found throughout Asia.
4. *Buthotus/Hottentotta*—natural habitat is in the Southern part of Africa extending up to Southeast Asia.
5. *Tityus*–Central and Southern America and the Caribbean regions are the natural habitat.

6. *Leiurus*—occurs in the Northern part of Africa and the Middle East.
7. *Androctonus*—present in Northern Africa and parts of Southeast Asia.
8. *Centruroides*—occurs in most parts of America, Mexico and the Caribbean regions.

B. *Hemiscorpius* species—also lethal species. Not too commonly found.

In India, several scorpion stings are endemic in Western Maharashtra, Karnataka, Andhra Pradesh, Saurashtra and Tamil Nadu, mainly involving the *Mesobuthus tamulus* species. Higher incidence of scorpion stings during the summer months is attributed to the increased agricultural activities.

Pathophysiology

Scorpions generally do not hunt for their prey, but wait for it. They are generally active only in the nights and try to avoid light during the daytime by hiding in cracks and crevices. Hence, the human stings occur, when they are disturbed and most of the stings occur on the hands and feet.

The stinger is located in the tail and the striated muscles in it allow the scorpion to regulate the amount of venom that is injected into the prey. The scorpion grasps the prey with its pincers, lifts its tail over its body in an arching action and drives the stinger with the venom into the prey. It can repeatedly sting the same prey and the amount of venom injected varies from 0.1 to 0.6 mg.

The venom glands are located on the tail, lateral to the tip of the stinger. The glands are lined by two types of tall columnar cells, one of which produces the venom, while the other produces mucus. The venom is an antigen containing water soluble, heterogenous mixture, which is composed of antigens that act on various end points. It has varying amounts of neurotoxin, nephrotoxin, cardiotoxin, hyaluronidase, serotonin, tryptophan, hemolytic toxin and cytokine releasers. The venom acts on the sodium channels to alter their conduction rates resulting in prolonged neuronal activity with resultant nerve hyperactivity. This effect is seen in the somatic as well as the cranial nerve endings. The end organ effects are secondary to the excessive neuronal excitation. The autonomic hyperexcitation results in the cardiopulmonary effects, while the pain associated with scorpion stings is secondary to the serotonin present in the venom. The neurotoxin of the scorpion venom is more toxic than that of snake venom and its LD50 has been shown to be 10 fold more than that of cyanide.

The neurotoxin is the most potent and causes impairment in the conduction of the heart, muscles and nerves due to the altered ionic permeability in the neurons. Due to the repeated firing, there occurs neuronal over excitation, release of excessive neurotransmitters like epinephrine, acetylcholine, glutamate and aspartate. The potassium channels are also blocked resulting in delayed recovery of the action potential. The binding of these neurotoxins to the host sites is reversible. It can be inactivated by reagents that break the disulfide bridges that give the neurotoxin its stability, thus causing unfolding of the toxins and its subsequent inactivation.

Children are more at risk from the lethality of the scorpion toxin due to their lower body weight, thus have more severe reactions and rapid progression of the symptoms due to the larger ratio of the venom to the body weight.

Symptoms

Symptoms vary depending on the duration between sting and presentation at the health facility. Hence, it is essential to check the exact time of envenomation, if possible along with a description of the scorpion species. Patients present with severe pain and paraesthesias. Nausea and vomiting may occur.

Stings on the head and neck result in quicker absorption into the central nervous system (CNS) via the circulation with quicker onset of symptoms. Local symptoms can progress to systemic symptoms rapidly, within 5 minutes to 4 hours after the sting and symptoms can persist for 10–48 hours. An 'autonomic storm' of symptoms is evoked, which is related to the transient parasympathetic followed by the prolonged sympathetic stimulation phase.

Signs

1. Local:
    - Swelling

- Hyperesthesia
- Tap test positive
- Macule/papule at site
- Lymphangitis
- Profuse sweating all over—'skin diarrhea'
- Effects secondary to release of kinins and slow-reacting substances (SRS).

2. Neurological:
   - CNS—altered consciousness
   - Abnormal behavior
   - Ataxia
   - Paresthesias in all four limbs
   - Parasympathetic—bronchoconstriction
   - Bradycardia
   - Hypotension, salivation
   - General weakness, miosis
   - Sympathetic—hyperthermia
   - Arrhythmias
   - Tachycardia, tachypnea
   - Hyperexcitability
   - Mydriasis.
3. Cardiovascular:
   - Early signs: hyperdynamic followed by hypodynamic phase (renin and catecholamine mediated)
   - Tachycardia is more than 130 bpm, hypertension
   - Apical pansystolic murmur
   - Toxin induced myocarditis—biventricular dysfunction
   - Cardiogenic shock.
4. Respiratory:
   - Tachypnea
   - Pulmonary edema—hemoptysis

- Respiratory failure secondary to alveolar hypoventilation, diaphragmatic collapse and bronchorrhea.

5. Gastrointestinal:
   - Hypersalivation—thick ropy saliva
   - Dysphagia
   - Gastric hyperdistension
   - Acute pancreatitis
   - Toxic hepatitis.
6. Allergic:
   - Urticaria
   - Angioedema
   - Bronchospasm
   - Anaphylaxis.
7. Hematological:
   - Platelet aggregation due to catecholamine stimulation
   - Disseminated intravascular coagulation (DIC) and massive hemorrhage due to toxin-mediated defibrination.
8. Genitourinary:
   - Decreased renal plasma flow
   - Acute tubular necrosis due to toxin
   - Priapism due to secondary cholinergic stimulation
   - Renal failure.
9. Metabolic:
   - Hyperglycemia due to hepatic glycogenolysis, pancreatitis and insulin inhibition
   - Electrolyte imbalance
   - Lactic acidosis.

Scorpion stings are diagnosed by a quartet of symptoms:

1. Extreme restlessness, flailing limbs and facial grimacing.
2. Mydriasis nystagmus.
3. Hypersalivation.
4. Dysphagia.

Time of onset of symptoms—within few minutes up to 5 hours after the sting. Signs may persist for up to 24–72 hours after the sting. No definite sequence of progression of the signs, hence predicting the outcome is extremely difficult.

Grading

The neurological predominance and non-neurological predominance as given in Tables 11.1 and 11.2.

Table 11.1: Neurological predominance

Grade	Symptoms and signs
1	Local pain or paresthesia at sting site
2	Pain or paresthesia at site distant from sting also found
3	Cranial nerve or somatic neuromuscular dysfunction
4	Both cranial nerve and somatic dysfunction present

Table 11.2: Non-neurological predominance

Grade	Symptoms and signs
Mild	Local signs only
Moderate	Ascending local signs or mild systemic signs
Severe	Life-threatening systemic signs

Laboratory Investigations

1. Complete blood count (CBC)—may show immediate leukocytosis and evidence of hemolysis in stings caused by particular species.
2. Blood glucose levels—hyperglycemia due to pancreatic insufficiency or hypoglycemia due to persistent vomiting.
3. Serum electrolytes—in patients with vomiting, diarrhea, hyersalivation, etc.
4. Coagulation parameters, partial thromboplastin time (PTT), activated partial thromboplastin time (APTT), international normalized ratio (INR)—to rule out DIC.
5. Renal function tests—to evaluate the renal functions.
6. Creatine kinase—in case of rhabdomyolysis.
7. Urinalysis—hemoglobinuria may be noted in cases of rhabdomyolysis.

8. Liver function tests—to evaluate the hepatic functions.
9. Arterial blood gas (ABG)—in case of respiratory distress.
10. Chest X-ray—essential in patients with respiratory symptoms. Evidence of unilateral pulmonary edema may be seen due to increased vascular permeability.
11. Electrocardiography (ECG)—reveals rhythm disturbances, commonly sinus tachycardia. Other disturbances such as QTc prolongation, ST changes, T-wave inversion, bundle branch block, first-degree conduction block, etc. ECG abnormalities found in majority of envenomated children.
    a. Arrowhead T-waves: acute injury (similar to Ashoka trees).
    b. Prolonged QTc and the conduction defects usually normalize within a week, while the T-wave inversion could persist for few weeks.
    c. Low voltage, wide QRS complexes, tachycardia and hemiblock, marked ST-segment depression, if persistent, indicate a poor prognosis.
12. Echocardiogram—has multiple uses.
    a. Myocardial compromise can be evaluated.
    b. Global biventricular hypokinesis with decreased left and right ventricular ejection fraction, which usually returns to normal values in 4–8 days.
    c. Normal left ventricular functions correlates with normal cardiopulmonary functions.
    d. Serial echo is useful to follow-up towards recovery, as noted by normalization of left ventricle (LV) wall function or deterioration towards development of cardiomyopathy.
13. Color Doppler—may show evidence of mitral incompetence secondary to venom-induced dilated cardiomyopathy.

Treatment

Emergency management:

1. Assess the ABCs and stabilize the patient.
2. Grade the severity of the scorpion sting.
3. Decide regarding hospitalization based on the Hector hospitalization score:

a. Priapism: +3.
b. Vomiting: +2.
c. Systolic BP greater than 160: +2.
d. Corticosteroid administered: +2.
e. Temperature greater than 38°C: +1.
f. Heart rate is greater than 100 bpm: +1.

Total score ≥ = 2: hospitalization required.

Local Treatment

1. Oral extraction of the sting contraindicated.
2. Use ice bags to reduce pain and slow venom absorption by vasoconstriction.
3. Immobilize the affected part in a functional position to delay venom absorption.
4. Calm and counsel the patient to decrease the heart rate and blood pressure (BP), which will also delay venom absorption.
5. An extractor may be used to deliver negative pressure of 1 atm at the sting site, may be useful to remove the venom.
6. Apply a topical anesthetic to decrease the paresthesia.
7. Administer local wound care and a topical antibiotic ointment.
8. Administer injection tetanus toxoid.

Systemic Treatment

1. Ensure that airway, breathing and circulation is established and maintained.
2. Monitor the vital signs; heart rate, respiratory rate (RR), BP and pulse oximetry.
3. Administer supplemental oxygen to ensure adequate tissue oxygenation.
4. Intravenous (IV) fluids—rapid in case of shock (20 mL/kg) and in maintenance doses in cases of vomiting, diarrhea, hypersalivation, sweating, etc.
5. If hyperdynamic circulatory changes are noted: administer combination of alpha-1 and beta-1 blockers or nitrates, which will combat myocardial ischemia and hypertension. Studies

in India have shown the better response of administration of prazosin + antivenom, wherein the requirement of the antivenom has been shown to be lesser with better patient outcome.

6. In case of pulmonary edema without hypotension—administer diuretics.
7. In case of massive pulmonary edema requiring rapid volume reduction, administering sodium nitroprusside as a vasodilator infusion is essential (Fig. 11.1).
8. For hypodynamic cardiac changes, administer an afterload-reducing agent like nifedipine, hydralazine or angiotensin-converting enzyme (ACE) inhibitors. Captopril (ACE inhibitor) improves cardiogenic shock as well as the pulmonary edema.
9. In case of resistant hypotension, dobutamine (5–20 μg/kg/min) is preferred for its inotropic effects as dopamine has catecholamine like actions and may aggravate the cardiac damage.
10. Atropine is useful for countering the parasympathomimetic effects.

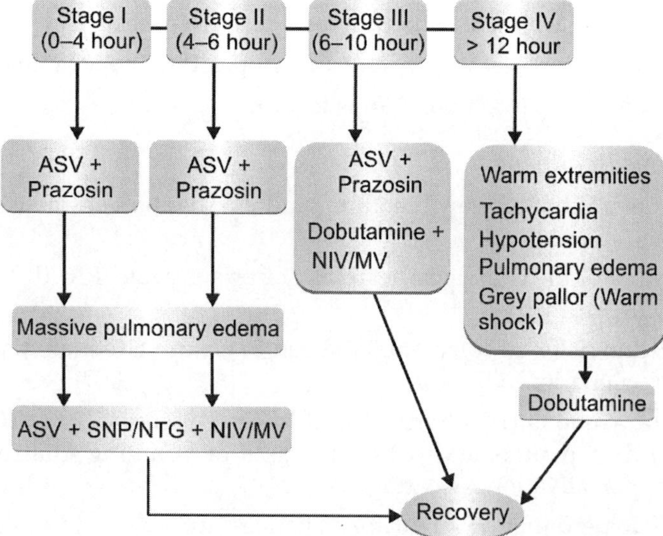

Fig. 11.1: Algorithm for treatment of scorpion stings. ASV, anti-scorpion venom; NIV, non-invasive ventilation; MV, mechanical ventilation; SNP, sodium nitroprusside; NTG, nitroglycerine.

11. Continuous pump infusion of barbiturates for excessive motor activity.
12. Use of antivenom: Scorpion antivenom is usually species specific. One species antivenom will have limited effect on another species. Antivenom decreases the level of the circulating unbound venom within a few hours, but does not act upon the toxin, which has already been bound to the receptors. Anaphylactic reactions can be decreased by skin testing. Dilute 0.1 mL of antivenin with sodium chloride in a 1:10 dilution and administer 0.2 mL of this solution intradermally. If a wheal appears within 10 minutes, it indicates hypersensitivity. However, the adverse effects are small in comparison with the positive effects that the antivenin can have especially if administered early during treatment. Hence, it is recommended to use the antivenom without doing a skin test.
13. In India, since the year 2002 the non-specific antivenom F(ab)2 SAV is available for clinical use, being the product of the Haffkine Biopharma company. 30 mL dose is usually sufficient to neutralize the effect of each sting, which could inject up to 1.5 mL of the venom into the body. However, in cases of severe stings more doses of the antivenom may be essential.
14. In case of hypersensitivity reactions, administer steroids.

Complications

- Persistent paresthesias
- Seizures
- Renal failure
- Dilated cardiomyopathy
- Rhabdomyolysis
- Respiratory arrest
- Pulmonary edema
- Pancreatitis
- Cardiac arrest.

Prognosis

Best results are seen, if appropriate supportive and specific treatment is administered early within 2 hours of the scorpion sting. Children usually take a longer time to recover and need to be closely monitored especially for the initial 48 hours.

Cause of Death

- Cardiovascular collapse
- Ventricular arrhythmias
- Respiratory failure
- Renal failure
- Cardiac arrest
- Fulminant seizures.

Fatality rate is less than 2%–4%.

SUGGESTED READING

1. Bawaskar HS, Bawaskar PH. Scorpion sting. JAPI. 2012;60.
2. Cheng D. Scorpion sting. envenomation.www. medscape.com [Accessed October, 2010].
3. Kleigman RM, Behrman RE, Jenson HB, et al. Nelson Textbook of Pediatrics, 18th edition. Elsevier Health Sciences Division; 2007.

12

Chapter

Spider Bite

SPIDER BITE ENVENOMATION

There are at least 20,000 species of spiders in the world, all of which are poisonous. They use this poison to kill their prey. However, the poison produced by most varieties are not too potent, their fangs are not too strong nor they are long enough to pierce the human skin and inject the venom in sufficient amounts as to cause a severe reaction.

There are four major varieties of spiders that are dangerous to the human species. These are:

1. Black widow spider: By far the most poisonous spiders. They have black shiny bodies with a red hourglass mark on the underside. They are small and shiny and prefer warm climates and dark quiet places like unused garages, meter boxes and unused furniture.
2. Brown recluse spider: These are orange-yellow to brown in color and have a violin-shaped mark on the body. They measure about 1 inch in length and are found in warm dry climates. They prefer undisturbed areas like basements, closets, attics, door frames and corners.
3. Hobo spider: Medium sized, brown in color with some markings on the skin.
4. Yellow sac spider: Pale insects, greenish tan or light brown in color. Their front legs are longer than the others and they build sac-like tubes in leaves, under logs and in shrubs, instead of weaving webs.

Symptoms and Signs

1. Intense burning pain, itching, swelling and redness at the site of the bite. In case of black widow bites, double sting marks may be visible at the site.
2. Cramping pain and intense muscle rigidity especially on the back, shoulders and chest.
3. Sometimes, especially with the brown recluse bites, there may be a deep purple area around the bite, surrounded by a whitish ring and an outer larger red ring. This can help in diagnosing the species of the spider that had caused the bite.
4. Headache, severe myalgia and dizziness.
5. Rash and itching.
6. Restlessness and anxiety, commoner with the black widow bites.
7. Excess salivation and epiphora.
8. Excessive sweating.
9. Weakness, tremors or paralysis of the limbs, especially lower limbs, which is common with the black widow bites.
10. Occasionally nausea or vomiting, is common with the brown recluse bites.
11. Anaphylactic shock can occur in rare cases.

Treatment

1. Reassure the child, while at the same time the attendant should also remain calm and composed.
2. Wash the area thoroughly with soap and water.
3. Place an ice pack or a cold towel to the area of the bite.
4. Administer paracetamol or acetaminophen to decrease the pain.
5. Administer antihistamine, chlorpheniramine maleate to decrease the signs of itching and local redness.
6. Administer tetanus prophylaxis.
7. Intravenous (IV) fluids may be administered in case of severe anaphylaxis.
8. Epinephrine to be given in case of severe anaphylaxis. Use the IV route in case of signs of peripheral circulatory collapse.

9. In case of severe muscle spasms, administer benzodiazepines.
10. In case of black widow bites, if the patient has uncontrolled hypertension seizures or severe symptoms, it may be essential to administer antivenin.

Prognosis

All symptoms resolve over 2–3 days. Death is rare, but could occur in younger children and in those with multiple bites. Bites from brown recluse could turn necrotic and ulcerate, which usually heal over 1 week. Occasionally, skin grafting is required and scars may remain in 10%–15% of cases.

SUGGESTED READING

1. Kleigman RM, Behrman RE, Jenson HB, et al. Nelson Textbook of Pediatrics, 18th edition. Elsevier Health Sciences Division; 2007.
2. Spider bite. www.childrenscolorado.org [Accessed October, 2012].
3. Spider bites. www.seattlechildrens.org [Accessed October, 2012].
4. The Children's Hospital of Philadelphia. Spider bites. www.chop.edu [Accessed October, 2012].

V

Section

Miscellaneous

13

Chapter

Button Battery Ingestion

INGESTION OF BUTTON BATTERIES

Button batteries are small, usually flat and round batteries that are commonly used in several electronic gadgets, toys, watches, clocks, hearing aids, torches, etc. They are easily removable from their socket and can be an attractive item for curious children to mouth. The sequelae are usually benign and have favorable outcomes.

Pathophysiology

Disc batteries vary in diameter from 7.9 to 23 mm and weigh anything from 1 to 10 g. The usual size, which is commonly swallowed are the batteries, which are around 10–11 mm, followed by the 20 mm batteries.

The batteries are made up of cadmium, silver, manganese, lithium, sulfur dioxide, zinc, etc. which are the constituents of the anode and the cathode. The case is usually made of copper, brass or steel. The battery contains sodium or potassium hydroxide, which facilitates the electrochemical reaction to occur through the separator (Fig. 13.1).

The plastic grommet insulates the anode from the cathode and prevents the passage of the electric current. Upon removal of the

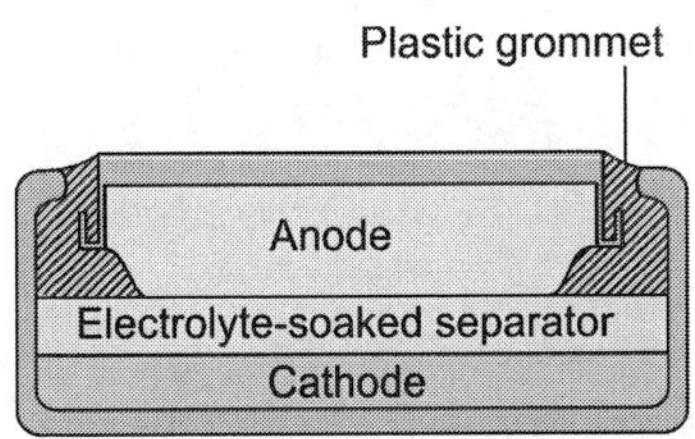

Fig. 13.1: Cross-section of a disc battery

grommet, the contact between the anode and the cathode is made, which results in the production of metal oxide at one end and reduction back to the metal at the other end, due to which the conductive current flows between the two ends.

The commonly ingested batteries are the lithium cells, which account for over 90% of the ingested batteries. They usually do not cause any problem and slide through the gastrointestinal tract (GIT), but cause difficulties if they get lodged, especially in the esophagus. The damage can occur fairly rapidly, as fast as within 2–2½ hours following ingestion.

Due to the current flowing through the battery, there is production of sodium hydroxide, which can result in necrosis due to liquefaction of the surrounding tissues. The amount of electricity generated depends on the battery voltage. The 20 mm lithium batteries are 3 V and generate more current than the 1.5 V, due to more sodium hydroxide production. Severe esophageal burns and perforation can occur, especially adjacent to the negative pole, which is the flat surface without any imprint on it. Despite laparoscopic removal of the battery, the residual alkali in the tissues can cause persistent tissue damage. The weak tissues of the esophagus can be easily damaged by any further trauma (Fig. 13.2).

Symptoms

Children below 4 years are common age group in whom this occurs.

Disc batteries are usually ingested immediately after removal from the gadget, hence the act of swallowing may be observed by elders around. Batteries discarded or those kept lying around with

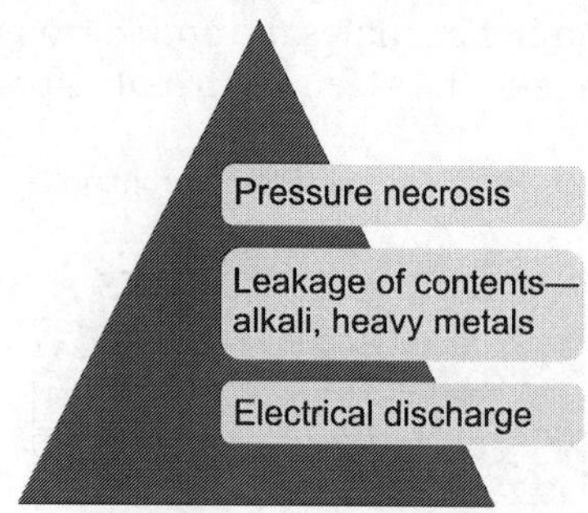

Fig. 13.2: Pathophysiology

intention to use are the most likely to be swallowed. Slightly older children may remove the battery from their toys, shoes, books, musical greeting cards, hearing aids, etc. and unwittingly swallow them after placing in the mouth.

Most often, the ingestion is asymptomatic, especially when it has passed down the esophagus, it is then excreted within 2–7 days in the stools. Occasionally, skin rashes may be noted, which is due to hypersensitivity, usually to the nickel batteries. About 10% of the children complain of minor GI symptoms like vomiting, which may be blood tinged, abdominal pain, greenish-colored stools, fever, rashes or very rarely present with difficulty in breathing. Occasionally, there maybe increased salivation, retrosternal discomfort.

Signs

No specific confirmative findings.

Common signs include:

- Increased salivation—black flecks in saliva
- Pyrexia
- Dysphagia
- Hematemesis
- Refusal of feeds
- Airway obstruction
- Abdominal tenderness
- Hematochezia.

Some types of cells, particularly those containing mercuric oxide, fragment in the stomach more easily than the others, hence cause more signs of GI irritation.

Investigations

X-ray of the abdomen is of utmost importance to confirm the presence and the location of the disc battery. They can be easily mistaken for a coin, but it is usually more rounded than the coin and has a step off at the junction of the cathode and anode. Radio-opaque droplets in the gut are visible in case of battery disintegration, especially the mercury containing cells. Batteries seen in the esophagus at initial examination, may spontaneously pass in the stomach due to the peristaltic movements.

Serum mercury levels: to be measured when there are clinical signs of mercury toxicity.

Treatment

1. Secure the airway, maintain adequate breathing and oxygenation and insert the intravenous (IV) access.
2. Maintain the patient nil orally and complete the radiological examination to note the site of the battery.
3. If the battery is in the esophagus and the patient has presented early within 2 hours of ingestion, flexible fiberoptic endoscopic removal is recommended.

   If the battery is in the esophagus and the patient has presented early within 2 hours of ingestion and no endoscopy facility is available, attempt the removal with the Foley catheter technique.
4. If the battery is past the esophagus and the patient is symptomatic, consider surgical removal.
5. If the battery is past the esophagus and the patient is asymptomatic, repeat the X-ray every week, while closely observe the stools for passage of the battery.
6. When the battery is ingested along with a magnet, it is essential to remove them endoscopically.
7. Chelation is indicated only when there are symptoms of mercury toxicity.
8. In cases where the battery is noted below the pylorus and delayed transit is possible, whole bowel irrigation, colon enema or cathartics may be useful to evacuate the battery.
9. Do not induce emesis, as this can cause regurgitation of the battery and impaction in the esophagus.

Algorithm for Treatment

The algorithm for treatment of disc battery ingestion is shown in the Figure 13.3.

Complications

1. Esophageal perforations.
2. Tracheoesophageal fistula.

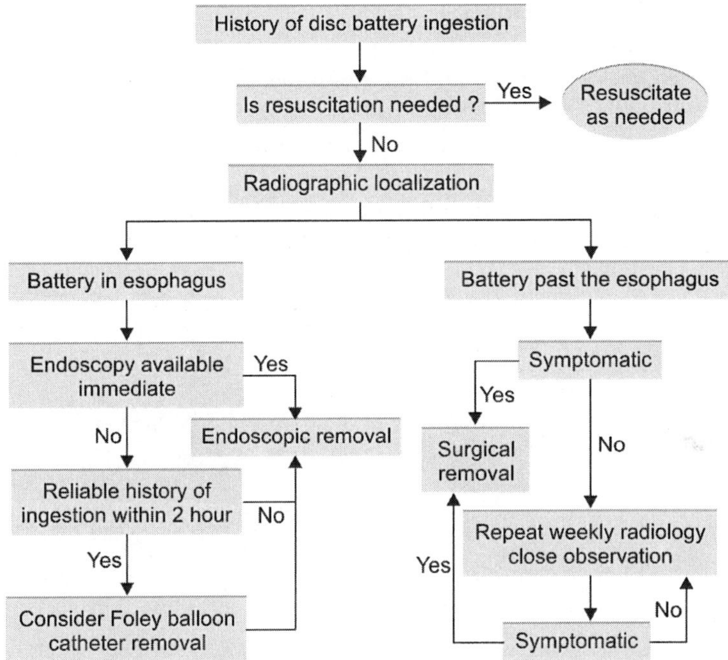

Fig. 13.3: Algorithm for treatment of disc battery ingestion

3. Esophageal stricture.
4. Recurrent laryngitis.
5. Vocal cord paralysis.
6. Tracheal stenosis.
7. Tracheomalacia.
8. Lung abscess.
9. Empyema.
10. Aspiration pneumonia.
11. Mediastinitis.
12. Pneumoperitoneum.

Prognosis

Usually recovery is uneventful in over 95%–97% of the cases. In others, the prognosis is related to the severity and the adequacy of early management.

SUGGESTED READING

1. Amanetidou V, Sofidiotou V, Fountas K. Button battery ingestion: the Greek experience and review of the literature. Pediatr Emerg Care. 2011;27(3):186-88.
2. Dire DJ. Disk battery ingestion. www.medscape.com [Accessed September, 2012].
3. Kleigman RM, Behrman RE, Jenson HB, et al. Nelson Textbook of Pediatrics, 18th edition. Elsevier Health Sciences Division; 2007.

14 Chapter Insect Stings

Insect stings, including bee stings are painful and can cause lethal effects in cases where the patient is allergic to the venom. Wasps and hornets are similar to bee stings and can cause allergic reactions in persons, who are allergic to bee stings. The wasps can sting several times and they usually do not leave their stinger behind.

SYMPTOMS

- Sudden intense pain at the sting site
- Redness, swelling
- Itching
- Burning sensation
- Difficulty in breathing
- Choking sensation.

SIGNS

1. Redness, erythema.
2. Wheal formation.
3. Swelling at site of bite.
4. Stings on the tongue can cause airway obstruction.
5. Signs of anaphylaxis: tachycardia, rapid thready pulse, peripheral cyanosis, angioedema.
6. Death can occur within 30 minutes, in severe anaphylaxis.

TREATMENT

1. Remove the stinger immediately. Do not squeeze, as this can inject more venom into the body.

2. Place an ice pack on the site of the sting. This will reduce the pain and the swelling.
3. Apply calamine lotion or antihistamine cream to decrease the itching.
4. Administer diphenhydramine, which will slow the anaphylactic reaction.
5. Ibugesic or paracetamol will decrease the pain associated with the sting.
6. In case of severe anaphylactic reaction, administer epinephrine.

Stings in the ear, nose or throat (ENT) can be fatal and must be immediately attended to by the ENT surgeon.

SUGGESTED READING

1. Canadian Food Inspection Agency. www.inspection.gc.ca/food/consumer-centre/fact-sheets/specific-products-and-risks/natural-toxins/eng [Accessed December, 2012].
2. Kleigman RM, Behrman RE, Jenson HB, et al. Nelson Textbook of Pediatrics, 18th edition. Elsevier Health Sciences Division; 2007.
3. Nguyen AT. Insect bites. www.emedicinehealth.com [Accessed October, 2012].
4. www.uogelph.ca/foodsafetynetweork/natural-toxins-fruits-and-vegetables [Accessed December, 2012].
5. www.enviromentalgraffiti.com/news-10-poisonous-fruits-and-vegetables [Accessed December, 2012].

15 Chapter Vegetable Poisons

According to the recommendations for a balanced diet, every person must consume at least 4–5 portions of vegetables and fruits per day in the diet. But do we know how safe the vegetables and fruits that we consume are? There are many poisons lurking in the foods we consume about which we must be aware and take steps to avoid or reduce their consumption (Table 15.1).

Table 15.1: Common vegetable and fruit poisons

Name of vegetable/fruit	Poison substance and location in the plant	Symptoms
Potato	Glycoalkaloid in stem and leaves, also in the potato, if left to turn green	Confusion, weakness, coma, death
Tomato	Glycoalkaloid in stem and leaves	Nervousness and disturbed stomach functioning
Rhubarb	Corrosive acid, as well as an unknown poison in its leaves	Severe pain abdomen
Apple	Cyanide in apple seeds	Several seeds are essential to produce symptoms of cyanide toxicity
Cherries	Prussic acid, a hydrogen cyanide derivative present in the seeds	Symptoms of cyanide toxicity
Plums, apricots and peaches	Leaves and seeds contain cyanide derivative	Eye pain, watery eyes, oral hypersecretions,

Contd...

Contd...

Name of vegetable/fruit	Poison substance and location in the plant	Symptoms
Bitter almonds	Cyanide present in the seeds	tightness in the chest
Castor beans	Ricin present in castor bean	Convulsions
Mushrooms	Poison in the entire mushroom	Severe abdominal cramps, vomiting, anaphylactic reactions

COMMON POISON SOURCES

Some of the common poison sources are listed in Table 15.2.

Table 15.2: Common poison sources

Product	Toxic agent
Paint thinner	Turpentine
Floor cleaner	Phenol
Toilet cleaner	Phenol
Iron tablets and syrup	Iron
Kumkum	Lead
Cough syrup	Theophylline
Bronchodilators	Theophylline
Anti-termite treatment solutions	Arsenic
Industrial effluent	Arsenic
Agricultural pesticides	Aluminium phosphide
Hypnotic and sedatives	Barbiturate
Muscle relaxant rubs and creams	Camphor
Camphor crystals or tablets	Camphor
Cold rubs, vicks, etc.	Camphor
Generator fumes	Carbon monoxide
Forest fires	Carbon monoxide
Paint remover	Methylene chloride—source of carbon monoxide

Contd...

Contd...

Product	Toxic agent
Solvent degreaser	Methylene chloride—source of carbon monoxide
Carpet and fabric cleaner	Ethylene glycol
Radiator fluid	Ethylene glycol
Toothpaste	Fluoride
Chrome and wheel cleaning product	Fluoride
Etching agents	Fluoride
Hajmola, churna	Fluoride
Industrial gas	Hydrogen sulfide
Kerosene oil	Kerosene
Paints	Lead
Ceramics	Lead
Gasoline	Lead
Painted toys	Lead
Battery	Mercury
Thermometer, barometer	Mercury
Photography materials	Mercury
Dental amalgam	Mercury
Perfumes	Inorganic mercury
Cosmetics	Inorganic mercury
Disinfectants	Inorganic mercury
Photocopying fluid	Methanol
Windshield washing fluid	Methanol
Industrial solvent	Methanol
Plant pesticides	Organophosphate compounds
Insect killers and repellents	Organophosphorus compounds
Oven cleaner	Phenol
Bleaching agents	Phenol
Mosquito coils	Pyrethrum

Contd...

Contd...

Product	Toxic agent
Anti-lice preparations	Pyrethrum
Pesticides for grains	Pyrethrum
Anti-scabies lotions	Pyrethrum
Chrysanthemum oil	Pyrethrum
Rodenticides	Yellow phosphorus, warfarin
Asprin solution	Salicylate
Antidepressants	Tricyclic agents
Wax polish	Turpentine
Tomato leaves and stem	Glycoalkaloids
Green potato, stem and leaves	Glycoalkaloids
Apple seeds	Cyanide
Castor beans	Ricin
Bitter almonds	Cyanide

SUGGESTED READING

1. Insect bites: An T Nguyen. www.emedicinehealth.com.
2. Kleigman RM, Behrman RE, Jenson HB, et al. Nelson Textbook of Pediatrics, 18th edition. Elsevier Health Sciences Division; 2007.

VI

Section

Preventive Measures

16 Chapter

Measures to Prevent Occurrence of Poisoning

MEASURES TO PREVENT OR REDUCE CHILDHOOD POISONING

Childhood poisoning is one of the most common reasons for admissions into hospital, especially in below 5 years age group. In this age group, the accidental poisonings are common occurrence and are mostly non-fatal. However, in the older children and adolescents, the toxin is intentionally ingested in most instances. These may be fatal depending on the amount of toxin ingested and may result in severe complications.

For the group with intentional ingestion, it is essential not only to administer the immediate treatment and give the life-saving support, but it is also essential to counsel these children and wherever needed, provide further psychiatric treatment to ensure that the child does not attempt nor repeat the episode in future. These children must be handled extremely carefully, as there always exists the likelihood of recurrence. The parents must be taken into confidence and also need to be counseled regarding the issues faced by the child. The issues range from peer group negativism, parental pressure for academic performance, school pressures and expectations, parental restrictions on activities, sibling rivalry, physical incapacities, etc. The child usually does not reveal the root cause of the problem and it is the duty of the treating physician to attempt to wean out the information or in case of extreme resilience, to involve a professional counselor to assist in the rehabilitation. These children also need to be regularly followed up after discharge from hospital, to evince any early signs of recurrence of the psychological imbalance. The parents must be counseled to ensure that the child does not have easy access to drugs and medications that may be easily misused. Also, it is mandatory to ensure that the child is engaged in sufficient activities to keep him adequately occupied and away from the thoughts of toxin consumption.

In the younger age groups, the accidental ingestion of toxins is extremely common. Here it is essential to draw up a protocol of treatment, while at the same time to follow simple steps, which can prevent the recurrence of the accident in future.

1. Do not refer to medications, tablets and capsules as candies, sweets or chocolates.
2. Keep all medications out of reach of children.
3. Keep all medications locked inside the child resistant cupboards.
4. Keep medications in the refrigerator in locked containers.
5. Ensure that all household cleaning agents, chemicals and pesticides are securely stored in locked areas.
6. Keep all cleaning agents, disinfectants and pesticides in their original containers and covers.
7. Dispose of unused or expired medications and household chemicals in appropriate manner.
8. Iron tablets and other herbal remedies can also be highly toxic, hence they need to be stored just as other medications are kept.
9. Ensure that all visitors and guests take care to secure their medications and dangerous substances and do not leave them around in easily accessible places like handbags, bedside, etc.
10. Cigarettes, alcohol and other narcotics can be highly toxic to children. Ensure that the ashtrays are kept empty and that the intoxicants are kept securely locked.

SUGGESTED READING

1. Hockey R. Childhood poisoning and ingestion. Injury Bulletin. 2000; No 60.
2. Kleigman RM, Behrman RE, Jenson HB, et al. Nelson Textbook of Pediatrics, 18th edition. Elsevier Health Sciences Division; 2007.

Index

Page numbers followed by *f* refer to figure and *t* refer to table, respectively.

A

B

C

D

J

K

L

M

Q

R

S

T

U

V

W

Y

Z